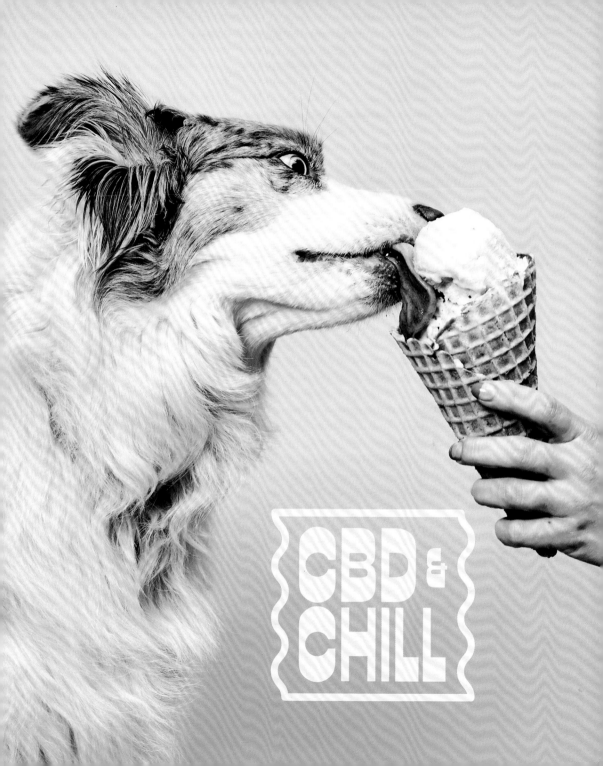

CBD &

75 Self-Care Recipes for Everyday Wellness

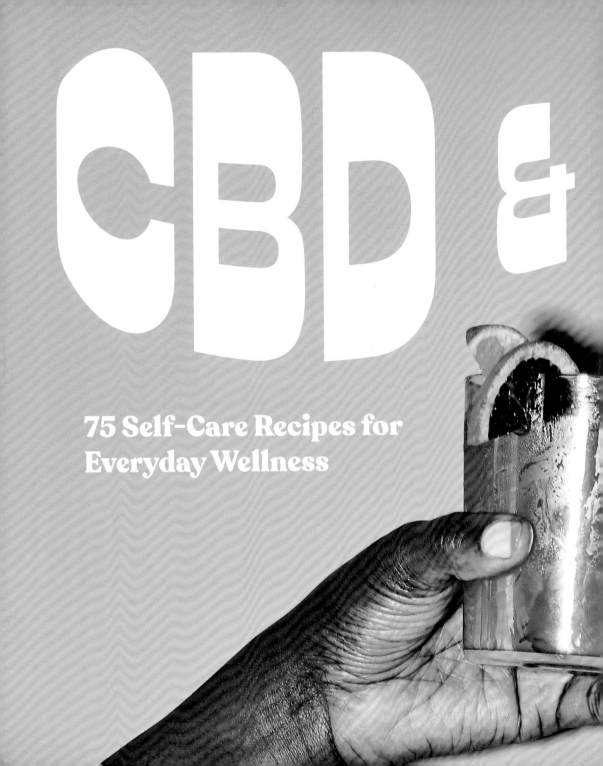

CHILL

TORI BODIN
· Founders
of Dazey ·
CHRIS TARELLO

SASQUATCH BOOKS
SEATTLE

PART II GO FOR THE GLOW

THE

A TO Z

OF

CBD

OUR JOURNEY WITH CBD

Both in our business and personal experience, we believe life should be enjoyed with "no bad daze." We make time for laughter, no matter how hectic our schedules, and we embrace our motto of "CBD & Chill" every day. At our core, we're natural beauty and remedy advocates with a profound passion for hemp, but we never take ourselves too seriously. After all, what's wellness if you can't acknowledge and appreciate the little mistakes in life? Before we founded Dazey, both of us were working in tech and we were stressed out (like an unmanageable level of stressed out). We needed to find something that would help us relax throughout the day and improve our focus and attention to detail. We needed to feel calm and friendly, but not sedated. A coworker recommended CBD.

It checked all the boxes: natural, nonpsychoactive, and discreet. We picked up a mint chocolate–flavored tincture at a natural food store; with daily use, we noticed a difference in how we approached our scope of work. We discovered a better sense of equilibrium between productivity and creativity, helping us feel less overwhelmed and anxious about approaching deadlines and never-ending inboxes. We discovered something that helped us manage our stress and kick ass at work, and we knew that this little cannabis compound was something special. Our passion for its benefits only grew as we continued to find relief over the following weeks and months.

This was early 2018, and over the course of that year, we tried about ten different tinctures. After growing tired of the mint chocolate flavor of the first tincture, we landed on our favorite from a small farm in neighboring Oregon. It was exactly what we were looking for: no artificial flavors, sweeteners, or other additives. It contained just hemp and coconut oil and had a pleasant, versatile taste. We got to know the farmers and understand their cultivation methods, educated ourselves on the legality of hemp in the United States, and became genuinely passionate about the product. One day it crossed our minds that, as young professionals with a trustworthy perspective, we may be uniquely qualified to introduce the benefits of CBD to our peers. We asked the farm if they would be open to letting us apply our marketing experience to the product and launch our own brand. They agreed and we enlisted our best friends, who are also incredibly talented designers, to bring our vision to life.

Inspired by the design and colors of California surf posters—evocative of sand and sea and stunning sunsets—the four of us spent nights and weekends creating brand concepts and building a story around West Coast wellness. Not too long after, we founded Dazey: a lifestyle brand that celebrates CBD for its ability to integrate seamlessly into our lives and our daily rituals.

Our mission is to destigmatize CBD in the workplace and in everyday life. We believe education is the foundation for understanding how CBD can become a part of your own rituals. We want hemp, a plant whose relationship status with the United States has remained "it's complicated," to be approachable and understood. We want to see friends sharing recipes and experiences with various applications and dosages. Since our launch, we've happily witnessed customers engaging with one another and with their communities, and we're constantly impressed with the leaders and advocates of this industry as a whole.

By the time this book is published, we'll be getting ready to celebrate Dazey's second anniversary. Our first year in business has been a wild ride: We've made new friends and exhibited at events like West Coast Craft and the Indie Beauty Expo. We launched in our favorite brick-and-mortar stores across the country and at online retailers like Fleur Marché (founded by two Goop alumni) and Urban Outfitters. We've partnered with Rachel's Ginger Beer, Seattle's famous ginger beer company, to create two incredible CBD-infused flavors, and we launched a clothing collaboration with Girl Gang the Label (check out our podcast episode with them!). We joined experiential stores like Re:store in San Francisco and Neighborhood Goods in Texas, both of which are pioneering the future of retail. We expanded into CBD-infused skin care and beauty—and now have published a book! We're incredibly grateful for it all and optimistic about what comes next.

We hope you'll love this book and the recipes inside, whether it's your first time with CBD or you're already a daily user. And we hope we can be your knowledgeable stewards to understanding the power of hemp both today and for years to come. After all, that's the secret to #NoBadDaze. Enjoy!

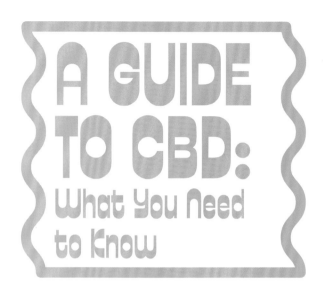

A GUIDE TO CBD: What You Need to Know

CBD is everywhere. You've seen it in coffee shops, boutiques, and drug stores. But what is it *exactly* and what should you be looking for? A lot of information is out there but digging up what's true and accurate on your own can be daunting. That's where we come in. We're going to be your guide to understanding the truth about CBD—how it interacts with your body, how to find the right CBD product for you, and how you can incorporate this natural adaptogen into your daily routine.

What Is It, *Exactly?*

Let's start with the basics. CBD (or cannabidiol) is a cannabinoid found in cannabis, the plant genus that includes hemp and marijuana. CBD can be smoked, vaporized, ingested, or applied topically. It's an increasingly popular ally for fighting stress, anxiety, inflammation, lack of focus, insomnia, and dry skin, to name a few. Scientists and researchers have discovered that CBD also has antioxidant and neuroprotective properties, promotes brain cell production, and maintains gut health.

Our most commonly asked question is, "Does CBD get you high?" And the answer is no. CBD has *zero* psychoactive effects. "But doesn't it come from the cannabis plant?" To answer this question and to understand the intricacies of CBD, we must first travel back in time to learn a bit more about the social, political, and medicinal history of cannabis.

A Brief History of Cannabis

Mentions of cannabis as a versatile plant date back to some of the oldest texts. In the year 570, a French queen was buried in hemp clothing, and Vikings used hemp in as early as 850 to outfit themselves. In 1533, King Henry VIII of England fined farmers if they did not grow hemp.[1] Evidence exists of nineteenth-century Western doctors prescribing cannabis for pain. In the early 1900s, you could even buy the plant in pharmacies! But the public and political opinion surrounding cannabis in the United States shifted in the early twentieth century with the release of films such as *Reefer Madness* and newspaper articles that painted the plant in a dangerous and damaging light. This was a direct backlash to the current social and political situation in the US. Between 1910 and 1920, the US saw a huge influx of Mexican immigrants looking for refuge from civil war.[2] These immigrants brought cultural habits of recreational cannabis use to the mainstream US. This was great for cannabis, and the plant became increasingly popular in places like California and Texas, but not everyone was on board. During the Great Depression, US politicians were looking for someone to blame, and immigrants and "their foreign substance" became the targets. Around this time, the term "marijuana" was coined to further associate cannabis with foreignness, and the plant's rich medicinal history went up in smoke.[3]

This propaganda and politicizing only grew in fervor with the Marihuana Tax Act of 1937,[4] a criminal law that imposed sanctions on those who sold, bought, or possessed marijuana. Hemp farmers took a huge hit during this time and were forced to change crops or face massive government taxation. This was a stark change from the US's historical sentiment on hemp. In the 1700s, American farmers in many colonies were required to grow hemp. The Declaration of Independence was drafted on hemp paper, and Abraham Lincoln used hemp seed oil to fuel the lamps in his home. In 1916, the United States Department of Agriculture (USDA) published findings that showed hemp produces four times more paper per acre than trees.[5] This fruitful history indicates that the passing of the Marihuana Act was a political move.

Even with the Marihuana Act's restrictions, hemp continued to gain recognition. In 1938, *Popular Mechanics* published a story about how hemp could be used in over twenty-five thousand products. In 1942, Henry Ford built an experimental car body made of hemp fiber that was ten times stronger than steel![6]

The final blow to cannabis came with Nixon's "War on Drugs" and his administration's signing of the Controlled Substances Act of 1970, which classified cannabis (hemp included) as a Schedule I drug, or a substance with "no known medicinal value," and transitioned oversight from the USDA to the Federal Drug Administration (FDA).[7]

The legal cannabis landscape was quite dreary until President Barack Obama signed the Agricultural Act of 2014 (a.k.a. the Farm Bill),[8] which defines industrial hemp as distinct from marijuana and authorizes institutions of higher education or state departments of agriculture in states that legalized hemp cultivation to regulate and conduct research and pilot programs.

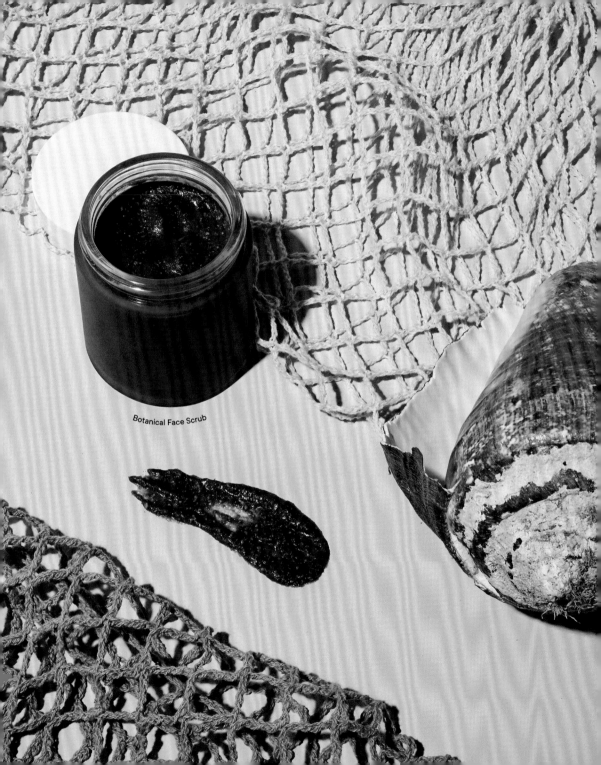

Botanical Face Scrub

Many farmers across the country (including ours!) were accepted into the pilot program and, just like that, hemp cultivation was back in the US. After almost eighty years, the US could once again start to regain the hemp knowledge and industry that was lost.

One of the biggest wins for hemp came with the passing of the 2018 iteration of the Farm Bill.[9] This bill removed the hemp plant, along with any of its seeds and derivatives, from the Controlled Substances Act as long as the hemp in question contains less than 0.3 percent THC. This was the most influential and positive legislation in the history of modern American hemp.

Today, we're living in a cannabis renaissance (cannabaissance?). The social stigmas of the past are beginning to melt away as states across the country legalize cannabis for medical and recreational purposes. The next decade will be revolutionary for cannabis. We're on the cutting edge—and we're happy to have you along with us for the ride.

Cannabis: Marijuana versus Hemp

Cannabis (or *Cannabis sativa*) is a genus of plants that includes marijuana and hemp. Although they're relatives, marijuana and hemp have distinct differences in their biology, appearance, and cultivation methods.

The most important difference between marijuana and hemp is the cannabinoids that each plant produces. Cannabinoids, the chemical compounds that cannabis plants secrete, offer a wide range of therapeutic benefits. When you consume cannabis, cannabinoids bind to different receptors throughout the body. More than one hundred cannabinoids have been identified, with many more waiting to be discovered; most exist in such minuscule amounts, however, that scientists have trouble identifying their exact influence on the body. Two of the most commonly occurring cannabinoids in cannabis plants are THC (or tetrahydrocannabinol), which is strongly psychoactive—the one that gets you high—and CBD (or cannabidiol), which is nonpsychoactive and soothing.

Marijuana is the high-inducing cannabis plant, carefully monitored to optimize its naturally occurring THC content. Its cousin, the hemp plant, is much more hardy, usually grown outdoors, and contains high CBD content and less than 0.3 percent THC. Between the roots, seeds, stalks, leaves, and flowers, hemp has thousands of applications, including extracting CBD for therapeutic purposes.

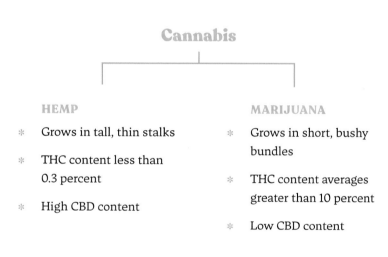

Cannabis

HEMP

* Grows in tall, thin stalks

* THC content less than 0.3 percent

* High CBD content

MARIJUANA

* Grows in short, bushy bundles

* THC content averages greater than 10 percent

* Low CBD content

Cannabinoids: THC versus CBD

Cannabinoids interact with a biological pathway inside your body called the endocannabinoid system, which regulates a variety of cognitive and psychological processes such as mood, memory, metabolism, and inflammation.

Two primary endocannabinoid receptors have been identified as CB1 and CB2. CB1 receptors are found primarily in the brain and are influenced by anandamide, a neurotransmitter responsible for pleasure, motivation, and hunger. This is the same neurotransmitter released during exercise that causes "runner's high." THC, extremely similar in molecular structure to anandamide, fits perfectly into CB1 receptors. This is why THC influences pleasure, motivation, and hunger, and makes you feel *hiiiigh*. CBD does not directly bind to CB1 receptors, but rather, indirectly inhibits them. This is why CBD can be used to reduce how high you feel after consuming THC as well as relieve psychological and mental stressors in the brain.

CBD also indirectly influences CB2 receptors, which exist primarily outside of the brain on white blood cells, in your tonsils, in your spleen, and throughout the rest of your body. The unbalanced functioning of CB2 receptors has been linked to virtually every type of human disease from cardiovascular, gastrointestinal, neurodegenerative, and autoimmune disorders to skin and bone ailments and even cancer. As CBD enters your bloodstream, it acts on CB2 receptors throughout your body to promote homeostasis, or stable equilibrium, of the endocannabinoid system. Research and clinical studies have found that this action on CB2 receptors produces anti-inflammatory and anticancer effects.

Other Cannabinoids, a.k.a. Cannabi-buddies

Besides CBD and THC, a number of other cannabinoids occur in hemp plants. These "cannabi-buddies" haven't received much recognition, but as more and more research is done on hemp, we're learning that even the most minute cannabinoids have an influence on how hemp extract affects our bodies.

Both THC and CBD (and CBC, on the following page) stem from the same precursor: CBG.[10] Think of CBG as the parent cannabinoid. During the six to eight weeks of the cannabis flowering cycle, an enzymatic reaction occurs that converts CBG to THC, CBD, or even minor cannabinoids like CBC. Although not often found in its isolated form, CBG appears to have many potential medical applications similar to CBD:

* Endocannabinoid receptors are prevalent in eye structures, and interestingly, CBG is thought to be particularly effective in treating glaucoma because it reduces intraocular pressure. It's also a powerful vasodilator and has neuroprotective effects to boot.[11]

* In animal experiments involving mice, CBG was found to be effective in decreasing the inflammation characteristic of inflammatory bowel disease.[12]

* In a 2015 study, CBG was shown to protect neurons in mice with Huntington's disease, which is characterized by nerve cell degeneration in the brain.[13]

* CBG is also showing great promise as a cancer fighter. Specifically, CBG was shown to block receptors that cause cancer cells to grow. In one such study, it inhibited the growth of colorectal cancer cells in mice, thereby slowing the spread of colon cancer. CBG inhibited tumors and chemically induced colon carcinogenesis, demonstrating a very exciting possibility for a cure for colorectal cancer.[14]

* European research suggests that CBG is an effective antibacterial agent, particularly against methicillin-resistant *Staphylococcus aureus* (or MRSA) microbial strains resistant to several classes of drugs. Since the 1950s, topical formulations

of cannabis have been effective in treating skin infections, but researchers at the time were unaware of the plant's chemical composition.[15]

* In a 2017 study, researchers showed that a form of CBG purified to remove delta-9-THC was a very effective appetite stimulant in rats. This may lead to an innovative nonpsychotropic therapeutic option for cachexia, the muscle wasting and severe weight loss seen in late-stage cancer and other diseases.[16]

* In a study that looked at the effects of five different cannabinoids on bladder contractions, CBG tested best at inhibiting muscle contractions, so it may become a tool to prevent bladder dysfunction disorders.[17]

CANNABICHROMENE (CBC)

CBC is a minor cannabinoid created through an enzymatic conversion from CBG. Not much is known about CBC in isolation, but preliminary research shows that it may carry pain-relieving properties, act as a potent anti-inflammatory agent, assist with digestive and gastrointestinal disorders, possess antibacterial and antifungal efficacy, and potentially contribute to the regeneration of brain cells.[18]

CANNABINOL (CBN)

A compound created when THC ages, CBN is nonpsychoactive. Have some old cannabis sitting in a drawer? Those nugs are undoubtedly packed with ripe CBN. Although current research on CBN is limited, studies have demonstrated that it may have powerful antibacterial, neuroprotectant, appetite-stimulating, and anti-inflammatory properties.

Some call CBN "the sleepy cannabinoid" because many people feel sedated after consuming aged cannabis, but this reputation might be misleading. As cannabis ages, not only is CBN created, but the terpene profile of the buds changes as well. Old cannabis contains more oxygenated, sedating terpenes. These terpenes, along with CBN's synergistic ability to increase the euphoric effects of THC, may be the true cause of sleepiness.[19] This wise and wrinkled cannabinoid just may be the greatest sleep aid since chamomile tea, but until more research is done, the only way to test how CBN affects you is to try it for yourself.

CANNABICYCLOL (CBL)

One of the lesser-known cannabinoids, CBL is a degradative product of CBN, similar to how CBN is a degradative product of THC. Most of the studies done on CBL have focused on its chemical structure, so little is known about its effects and potential benefits. We expect to see more research focusing on the effects of CBL soon.

Other Plant Components That Matter

CHLOROPHYLL

This molecule is responsible for giving cannabis its famous green pigmentation. Plants need chlorophyll to convert carbon dioxide and water, using sunlight, into oxygen and glucose. Hemp's chlorophyll packs a potent earthy aroma and flavor, and research shows that this little molecule displays anti-inflammatory properties[20] and can repair DNA cell damage.[21]

PLANT STEROLS

These naturally occurring fats, long considered an alternative health supplement, are thought to reduce cholesterol in humans. As a vote of confidence, the FDA allows for qualified health claims that credit sterol consumption with helping to keep blood pressure levels within a healthy range.

VITAMIN E

This common nutrient is important to vision, reproduction, and the health of your blood, brain, and skin. Vitamin E also has antioxidants that protect your cells against the effects of free radicals—molecules produced when your body breaks down food or is exposed to tobacco smoke and radiation. Foods rich in vitamin E include canola oil, olive oil, margarine, almonds, and peanuts. You can also get vitamin E from meats, dairy, leafy greens, fortified cereals, and, you guessed it, hemp extract.[22]

I hope we didn't lose you in the weeds there, no pun intended. The main takeaway is that CBD isn't the only powerful compound in hemp—a lot is going on inside our favorite stalky green plant. The more naturally occurring plant compounds you can get into your hemp extract, the more powerful its mood-balancing effects.

Dazey's full-spectrum oil, for example, contains CBD, THC (less than 0.3 percent), CBG, CBC, CBN, CBL, chlorophyll, plant sterols, and vitamin E. Talk about a party!

So now that you know (maybe more than you wanted to) about the inner workings of the hemp plant, let's talk about shopping for CBD—its different forms and methods of consumption, and what to look for on the label.

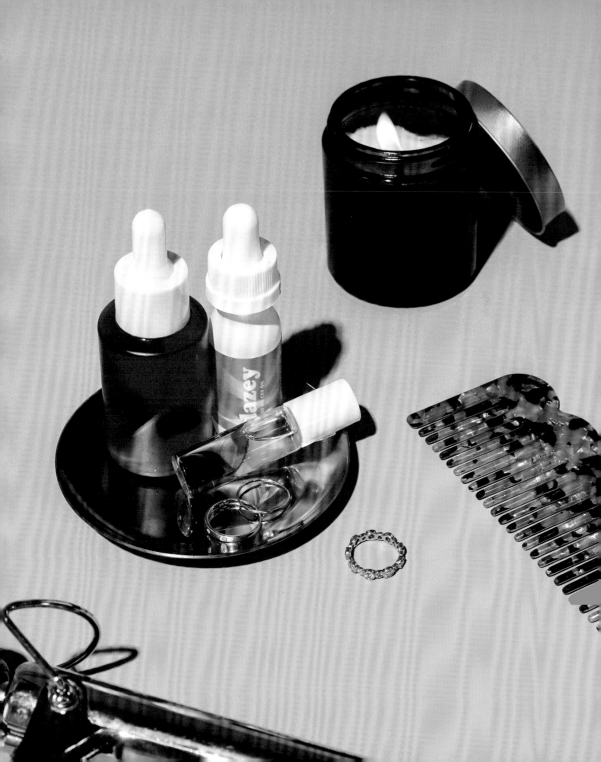

SHOPPING FOR CBD

You might have already started browsing online or at your favorite local retailers for CBD, only to find the product options overwhelming. At the time of this book's publication, there are still no official labeling requirements or guidelines for CBD products. While many of us earnestly want to give customers the right information, the lack of uniformity across the industry makes it difficult for customers to compare products apples to apples. Many companies don't even specify the type of CBD in their products or use misleading copy and marketing to convince consumers they're purchasing CBD when in reality, they're not. To make sure you're buying a quality product best aligned with your #CBDgoals, we recommend shopping from established marketplaces (see Directory, page 176) and looking for a few key product characteristics.

Ready? Let's get into it!

Breaking Down the Benefits

While there is no official categorization for types of CBD on the market, industry experts have adopted three terms to describe what's out there today: isolate, broad spectrum, and full spectrum.

Isolate CBD is stripped-down cannabidiol containing no other residual cannabinoids—zero percent THC and zero percent any other plant compound.

Broad-spectrum CBD means that a select number of compounds have been extracted from the plant. Every broad-spectrum product may contain different compounds, so read the contents on the label carefully and thoroughly.

Full-spectrum (or "whole plant") CBD utilizes all the therapeutic compounds found in hemp, including essential, monounsaturated, polyunsaturated, and saturated fatty acids; all naturally occurring hemp cannabinoids; terpenes; plant sterols; natural vitamin E; and chlorophyll. The interactive synergy of these compounds is known as the "entourage effect," a confluence of hemp goodness that increases the product's therapeutic power and medical benefits. In the United States, this type of CBD contains less than 0.3 percent THC.

Imagine a party with only one attendee. That's isolate. Imagine a small get-together where a few of your most fun friends canceled. That's broad spectrum. Now imagine a party with over one hundred guests happily mingling and sharing their collective consciousness. That's full spectrum.

Your personal preferences and needs will determine what type of CBD you choose. If you have a job that drug tests and your employer is not open to conversations on CBD consumption, you may want to go with isolate to avoid THC altogether. If you prefer a particular flavor or additive, you might find it in a broad-spectrum product.

If you're unsure and aren't concerned about trace amounts of THC, which will have zero psychoactive effects, we highly recommend a full-spectrum CBD. You'll experience the full therapeutic power of CBD this way.

Dispensaries versus CBD Retailers

Not all CBD is created equal. Based on where you're shopping, your options for CBD will be very different. For the most part, there are two main categories of stores that sell CBD. First, there are cannabis dispensaries. But it's rare to find hemp-derived CBD (less than 0.3 percent THC) in dispensaries, which are focused on selling marijuana-derived THC products unavailable at grocery stores and boutiques. So most of the CBD products sold in dispensaries contain enough THC to get you anywhere from mildly to "couch-lockingly" stoned. These products are labeled on a THC:CBD scale. A common ratio is 1:1, meaning the product contains equal parts THC and CBD. If you want to avoid even the slightest bit of psychoactive euphoria, be very cautious when shopping for CBD in dispensaries.

The second category of stores is everywhere else that sells CBD. The CBD you'll find at your favorite boutique or online retailer is required by federal law to contain *less than* 0.3 percent THC and therefore is defined as *hemp-derived*. This means you shouldn't get high or feel psychoactive effects, but to be hundo p, *always* ask to see testing results. All reputable CBD sellers are transparent about what exactly is in their oil, so whether you're shopping in person or online, do a quick Google search on the product first. An example of a product you would most definitely want to see testing results for would be one that claims to be full spectrum with zero percent THC. This is a clear contradiction to established industry definitions. At best, the product is poorly labeled, but at worst the manufacturer may be trying to mislead or confuse you.

The Importance of Testing Results

At Dazey, we post our testing results on our website and update them for every new batch of oil we create. We test for heavy metals, solvents, pesticides, cannabinoid content, and terpene profile to let our customers know exactly what they're getting. In the current unregulated state of the CBD industry, no company is *required* to post testing results, but any respectable and reputable CBD company will gladly make their findings available to consumers. As a consumer, it's imperative that you research before making a purchase. Make sure that you're getting what the label claims it contains and that your CBD has no nasty residual compounds from unethical production processes.

Here's what to look for in a product's Certificate of Analysis (COA):

* Purity: What is the product's cannabinoid concentration?

* No heavy metals: All extracted CBD should be tested to ensure that lead, mercury, arsenic, and cadmium levels are below the action limit, which is how a laboratory determines if a product passes or fails a test.

* No pesticides: Each state has different laws for pesticide testing. Although ingestion in small amounts may not cause immediate health issues, long-term exposure is linked to a variety of serious illnesses. When checking a COA, confirm that the report does not show "fail" for any tested pesticides.

* No residual solvents: Confirm that the product you're purchasing doesn't have excessive levels of residual solvents left behind from extraction.

Deciphering Labels

When you're reading a CBD product label, look for these key items:

BOTTLE COLOR: Sunlight can degrade CBD. High exposure to ultra-violet light and oxygen can rapidly break down organic matter like cannabinoids, so it's important to buy CBD products stored in dark or solid-color containers. Frosted glass is not ideal for storing CBD, but as long as you keep it in a cool, dark place, the oil should be okay.

POTENCY: It's essential to understand exactly how much CBD you're buying. First, determine the size of the container and the total milligrams of CBD in the product—the front label should clearly state this. Our oil comes in a fifteen-milliliter bottle with three different potencies to choose from: three hundred fifty milligrams, seven hundred milligrams, and one thousand milligrams. These amounts represent the total CBD content in milligrams per bottle. It can get confusing when you see two bottles of different sizes—one fifteen milliliters, the other thirty milliliters—that both contain one thousand milligrams of CBD. Both bottles contain the same total CBD content, but the thirty-milliliter product is less concentrated. In other words, you would need to take twice as much of the CBD in the thirty-milliliter bottle to equal the same dose from the fifteen-milliliter bottle.

FLAVORS OR ADDITIVES: It's important to know every ingredient in the product. Some CBD products, such as gummies, obviously will contain food ingredients such as pectin or syrups, and every CBD oil will be blended with some type of carrier oil, such as coconut, olive, or even hemp seed. However, with tinctures, additional additives might not be so obvious. For example, some CBD oil tinctures contain added flavors, sweeteners, preservatives, or essential oils. Read the ingredients panel carefully and confirm that the oil is safe for consumption—as opposed to topical use—and that it only contains ingredients you feel good about.

EXTRACTION METHOD: Two main methods are used to extract CBD oil today: CO_2 extraction, in which supercritical carbon dioxide pulls compounds from plants, and ethanol extraction, in which cannabis is soaked and then filtered to purge the alcohol from the extracted material. Ethanol extraction has been around for almost a century. There are detailed reports of ethanol-extracted cannabis tinctures being sold in apothecaries in 1937. CO_2 extraction was developed more recently and is also the backbone of the beer industry as the extraction method of choice for hops. Let's take a look at a few differences between the two methods:

* CO_2 preserves native terpenes and can be more cost-effective at scale. CO_2 is considered the cleanest, safest, and most cutting-edge method of extraction. For this reason, CO_2 processors are deemed to have more long-term viability and survivability in the market as more and more consumers care about how products are made.

* Ethanol has a lower price of entry, costs less to use, and produces a consistently high yield. Terpenes have a high probability of burning off, making this extraction method a viable choice for edibles and topicals.

Which method is better? It's up for debate—each has its pros and cons. It really comes down to what processors want in a final product. If taste and whole-plant compounds are a priority or if tinctures are the target product, CO_2 is the favored method.

TYPE OF CBD: Does this product contain isolate, broad-spectrum, or full-spectrum CBD (see page 17)?

ORIGIN: Where was the CBD sourced? Was the industrial hemp grown in the United States or imported? With the booming popularity of CBD, it isn't difficult to find domestically grown and extracted products. As more US-based players enter the CBD marketplace thanks to the 2018 Farm Bill, many international sellers are skirting the risk and forgoing importing to the States. That said, it's still possible to find imported CBD on some shelves as China and Canada are the top two producers of hemp, with the United States coming in third.

Understanding Terpenes

Aroma is tied to pretty much all of our experiences. Do you have a memory of a captivating plant? The way it smelled as the wind wafted its aroma under your nose? That scent was most likely a plant terpene—an aromatic chemical produced by many plants, including ginger, cinnamon, and hemp. Terpenes are the pungent oils that give cannabis its distinctive aroma and taste. There are over one hundred identified terpenes, and each strain of cannabis has a unique terpene profile, resulting in a unique user experience.

Because terpenes can interact with the other plant compounds present in cannabis, they're crucial to the entourage effect. Terpenes bind to the same receptors that CBD binds to and influence those receptors' chemical output.[23] So when it comes to efficacy, you should consider terpene, as well as cannabinoid, content. Most cannabis research has focused on cannabinoids, but recently scientists have begun to study and understand the intricacies and influences of terpenes.

Common terpenes found in cannabis include:

* Myrcene: Musky, earthy. Helps to encourage sleep and relaxation. Also found in mango, lemongrass, thyme, and hops.

* Limonene: Citrus. Relieves stress and elevates mood. Also found in fruit rinds, rosemary, juniper, and peppermint.

- Pinene: Pine. Reduces anxiety, increases alertness, and counteracts THC effects. Also found in pine needles, rosemary, basil, and dill.

- Caryophyllene: Peppery, woody. Relieves stress. Also found in black pepper, cloves, and cinnamon.

- Linalool: Floral. Enhances mood and relaxation. Also found in lavender.

- Humulene: Woody, earthy. Anti-inflammatory. Also found in hops, coriander, cloves, and basil.

- Ocimene: Sweet, herbal. Antibacterial, antifungal, and decongestant. Also found in mint, parsley, pepper, basil, mangoes, orchids, and kumquats.

- Terpinolene: Piney, floral, herbal. Relaxing. Also found in nutmeg, tea tree, apples, and lilacs.[24]

CBD Delivery Methods

CBD comes in all shapes and sizes. Literally. You can find CBD in almost anything these days, from tinctures and drinks to patches and suppositories. Determining how you will use CBD comes down to preference. For the purposes of this book, we'll be using CBD in a bottle with a calibrated dropper for precision, but there are plenty of options on the market.

TINCTURE: Any drop or spray form delivered directly into the mouth. This is the second-quickest way to absorb CBD and is definitely the most popular. Users can easily quantify their dose because tinctures usually have calibrated droppers. Tinctures also offer the most CBD per volume compared to other methods.

TOPICAL: The most cautious way to use CBD, this includes a wide array of products, from balms and lotions to rubs and patches. Topicals are effective in relieving muscle soreness but require liberal use to feel the effects, so a regular application can get expensive.

EDIBLE: Almost everything these days has a CBD variant. This is the tastiest way to dose, but the CBD in edibles takes longer to absorb through your digestive system.

VAPE/SMOKING: This is the fastest way to feel the effects of CBD, but it is difficult to control dosage. If you choose to vape your CBD, it's important that you find a reliable source. There have been numerous vaping-related illnesses and deaths from subpar or tampered products. The FDA has released this statement regarding vaping: "Consumers who choose to use any vaping related products should not modify or add any substances such as THC or other oils to products purchased in stores and should not purchase any vaping products, including those containing THC, off the street or from other illicit channels."[25]

If you're having trouble finding a product to suit your needs, take a look at the Directory on page 176, where we list a number of trusted sources and online retailers.

DOSING

Confused about what constitutes the right dose of CBD? You're not alone. Here's the important thing to remember: the appropriate dosage is completely personal. There's no "one size fits all" when it comes to CBD. Everyone processes cannabinoids differently based on body weight, metabolism, and unique endocannabinoid receptor characteristics. It's not as simple as getting a prescription from your doctor. It might take a lot of trial and error to find the perfect dose for the relief you're seeking. Here are a few questions to start you on your journey:

* What's your why?

    What do you want to get out of CBD? Determine what you're trying to solve with CBD.

* Be realistic.

    CBD is not a cure-all or an instant-fix product. It takes time, usually one to three weeks of consistent use, to discover the benefits of CBD. Your CBD journey is a marathon, not a sprint.

* Start slowly.

    In general, we recommend starting with a lower dose—ten to fifteen milligrams. But listen to your body—a slow start might not be right for you. The key to finding your perfect dosage is being present and making a conscious effort to track your intake. We lay out a recommended process for finding your ideal dose in our Weekly Dosing

Tracker on page 30. We also recommend using a journal to keep track of your daily CBD intake to pinpoint that sweet spot.

✳ Check your fear.

CBD is nontoxic and nonpsychoactive, and new users should not worry about taking too much. There are virtually no negative side effects to CBD use as long as you dose with a reasonable amount, such as five to thirty milligrams. Give CBD enough time to work by regularly dosing for days or sometimes weeks, depending on the person.

✳ Full spectrum for full benefits.

Even if you're new to CBD, go full spectrum. These products have the most active hemp compounds, allowing you to experience the power of the entourage effect—the powerful union of all the natural compounds hemp extract has to offer.

Okay, so now you're pumped and ready to dose. But how much is the right dose for you? Here's a good process to help you find out:

1   Avoid using any cannabis products for at least two days. This allows your body to return to its natural idle.

2   Be conscious. Ask yourself a few questions relating to your use case. If you're looking to balance your mood, consider: "How calm do I feel?" "How tolerant am I of others?" For inflammation, think about: "How easy is it to move?" "Is it hard to go about my normal day?"

3   Take five milligrams of CBD. This is most easily done with a tincture.

4   Wait forty-five minutes to one hour and then check in with yourself. Ask the same questions from step 2. If your answers haven't changed, take five more milligrams and repeat this step. When your answers have positively changed, you've found your lowest effective dose.

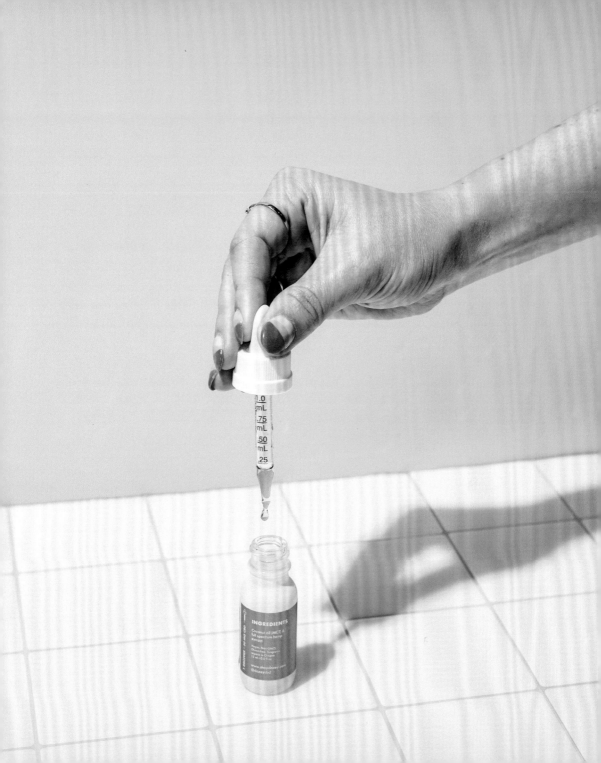

When it comes to frequency, again, this is going to be totally personal. You'll need to experiment by spacing out your dose over the course of many days or weeks and recording how you feel. We recommend taking a dose twice a day, about four to six hours apart to roughly maintain the effects of CBD throughout waking hours. Of course, there are many ways to consume, including microdosing and macrodosing.

Dosing: Micro & Macro

To understand microdosing, let's take a little trip back to where it all began. Dr. Albert Hofmann, a Swiss scientist responsible for creating and studying LSD in the mid-1900s, believed that acid could help people realize their full potential. He was also aware—from casual recreational use, no doubt—that at its full dose, LSD could inhibit a patient from completing daily tasks. So, to put some hard data behind his hypothesis, Hofmann began taking a daily microdose of LSD—just a fraction of what you'd need to experience a full trip, but enough to yield the subtler benefits of increased awareness and appreciation for one's surroundings.

Now, CBD oil is vastly different from LSD. CBD is a naturally occurring compound and does not produce psychoactive effects. But, as with Hofmann and his LSD, microdosing can help some users get the most benefit out of their CBD.

Remember that the endocannabinoid system manages and regulates processes like mood, metabolism, and inflammation. For someone using CBD, microdosing over the course of a day is especially useful for avoiding the peaks and pits of a fluctuating endocannabinoid system. By taking smaller doses more often, you can extend the potential benefits of CBD throughout an entire day, essentially maximizing and maintaining homeostasis for a longer period.

Managing chronic inflammation or pain is one of the best reasons for microdosing CBD. This method was popularized most recently by professional athletes, who must maintain peak performance through rigorous, inflammation-inducing activity. If you'd like to use CBD to manage a chronic issue, give microdosing a try.

MICRODOSING: Experimentation is your friend. Start by taking your lowest effective dose. Stay conscious and try to pinpoint the moment you start to feel the effects of CBD waning. This is your signal to take another dose. Remember, the timing here will be different for everyone; testing is the key. What you want to avoid is feeling any sedative effects. If you begin to feel sleepy, you've taken too much.

MACRODOSING: Another method of consuming CBD is macrodosing, the thicc twin of microdosing. The strategy here is to take double or triple your preferred dose to combat flare-ups of inflammation, anxiety, or insomnia. If you're using CBD to alleviate infrequent but severe symptoms, macrodosing could be a great option for you. Whenever you feel your symptoms coming on, take a double or triple dose and then listen to your body. In this case, it's okay to feel a mild sedative effect from CBD. The key is to focus on whether your macrodose is able to mostly alleviate your flare-up.

Weekly Dosing Tracker

You can find a digital copy of this dosing tracker on ShopDazey.com to use and keep with you as you fine-tune your dose.

Monday

MY MORNING DOSE WAS:

_____ mg

PRODUCT NAME:

_____

FORM:
- ☐ Food
- ☐ Beverage
- ☐ Tincture
- ☐ Topical

LAST NIGHT, I SLEPT:
- ☐ Great
- ☐ Good
- ☐ Okay
- ☐ Terrible

THIS MORNING, I FEEL:
- ☐ Excited
- ☐ Stressed
- ☐ Tired
- ☐ Happy
- ☐ In physical pain

MY EVENING DOSE WAS:

_____ mg

FORM:
- ☐ Food
- ☐ Beverage
- ☐ Tincture
- ☐ Topical

THIS EVENING, I FEEL:
- ☐ Excited
- ☐ Stressed
- ☐ Tired
- ☐ Happy
- ☐ In physical pain

Tuesday

MY MORNING DOSE WAS:

_____ mg

PRODUCT NAME:

_____

FORM:
- ☐ Food
- ☐ Beverage
- ☐ Tincture
- ☐ Topical

LAST NIGHT, I SLEPT:
- ☐ Great
- ☐ Good
- ☐ Okay
- ☐ Terrible

THIS MORNING, I FEEL:
- ☐ Excited
- ☐ Stressed
- ☐ Tired
- ☐ Happy
- ☐ In physical pain

MY EVENING DOSE WAS:

_____ mg

FORM:
- ☐ Food
- ☐ Beverage
- ☐ Tincture
- ☐ Topical

THIS EVENING, I FEEL:
- ☐ Excited
- ☐ Stressed
- ☐ Tired
- ☐ Happy
- ☐ In physical pain

Wednesday

MY MORNING DOSE WAS:

_____ mg

PRODUCT NAME:

_____

FORM:
- ☐ Food
- ☐ Beverage
- ☐ Tincture
- ☐ Topical

LAST NIGHT, I SLEPT:
- ☐ Great
- ☐ Good
- ☐ Okay
- ☐ Terrible

THIS MORNING, I FEEL:
- ☐ Excited
- ☐ Stressed
- ☐ Tired
- ☐ Happy
- ☐ In physical pain

MY EVENING DOSE WAS:

_____ mg

FORM:
- ☐ Food
- ☐ Beverage
- ☐ Tincture
- ☐ Topical

THIS EVENING, I FEEL:
- ☐ Excited
- ☐ Stressed
- ☐ Tired
- ☐ Happy
- ☐ In physical pain

Thursday

MY MORNING DOSE WAS:

_____ mg

PRODUCT NAME:

_____

FORM:
- [ ] Food
- [ ] Beverage
- [ ] Tincture
- [ ] Topical

LAST NIGHT, I SLEPT:
- [ ] Great
- [ ] Good
- [ ] Okay
- [ ] Terrible

THIS MORNING, I FEEL:
- [ ] Excited
- [ ] Stressed
- [ ] Tired
- [ ] Happy
- [ ] In physical pain

MY EVENING DOSE WAS:

_____ mg

FORM:
- [ ] Food
- [ ] Beverage
- [ ] Tincture
- [ ] Topical

THIS EVENING, I FEEL:
- [ ] Excited
- [ ] Stressed
- [ ] Tired
- [ ] Happy
- [ ] In physical pain

Friday

MY MORNING DOSE WAS:

_____ mg

PRODUCT NAME:

_____

FORM:
- [ ] Food
- [ ] Beverage
- [ ] Tincture
- [ ] Topical

LAST NIGHT, I SLEPT:
- [ ] Great
- [ ] Good
- [ ] Okay
- [ ] Terrible

THIS MORNING, I FEEL:
- [ ] Excited
- [ ] Stressed
- [ ] Tired
- [ ] Happy
- [ ] In physical pain

MY EVENING DOSE WAS:

_____ mg

FORM:
- [ ] Food
- [ ] Beverage
- [ ] Tincture
- [ ] Topical

THIS EVENING, I FEEL:
- [ ] Excited
- [ ] Stressed
- [ ] Tired
- [ ] Happy
- [ ] In physical pain

Saturday

MY MORNING DOSE WAS:

_____ mg

PRODUCT NAME:

_____

FORM:
- [ ] Food
- [ ] Beverage
- [ ] Tincture
- [ ] Topical

LAST NIGHT, I SLEPT:
- [ ] Great
- [ ] Good
- [ ] Okay
- [ ] Terrible

THIS MORNING, I FEEL:
- [ ] Excited
- [ ] Stressed
- [ ] Tired
- [ ] Happy
- [ ] In physical pain

MY EVENING DOSE WAS:

_____ mg

FORM:
- [ ] Food
- [ ] Beverage
- [ ] Tincture
- [ ] Topical

THIS EVENING, I FEEL:
- [ ] Excited
- [ ] Stressed
- [ ] Tired
- [ ] Happy
- [ ] In physical pain

Sunday

MY MORNING DOSE WAS:

_____ mg

PRODUCT NAME:

_____

FORM:
- [ ] Food
- [ ] Beverage
- [ ] Tincture
- [ ] Topical

LAST NIGHT, I SLEPT:
- [ ] Great
- [ ] Good
- [ ] Okay
- [ ] Terrible

THIS MORNING, I FEEL:
- [ ] Excited
- [ ] Stressed
- [ ] Tired
- [ ] Happy
- [ ] In physical pain

MY EVENING DOSE WAS:

_____ mg

FORM:
- [ ] Food
- [ ] Beverage
- [ ] Tincture
- [ ] Topical

THIS EVENING, I FEEL:
- [ ] Excited
- [ ] Stressed
- [ ] Tired
- [ ] Happy
- [ ] In physical pain

THE FUTURE OF HEMP AND CBD

While this book is focused on CBD, hemp has many other capabilities as one of the most versatile plants and the world's oldest domesticated crop. Rope, clothing, shoes, paper, textiles, food, bioplastics, concrete, insulation, biofuel—hemp can create them all. And that's only scratching the surface! By utilizing its roots, stalks, leaves, flowers, and seeds, we can find thousands of applications for hemp that could replace many nonbiodegradable materials.

CBD has incredible potential to reduce our reliance on pharmaceuticals. At this time, much is still unknown about CBD's medical benefits and long-term effects, but what we do know is incredibly promising.

Hemp can help reduce our reliance on fossil fuels and is a 100-percent biodegradable replacement for plastic. Hemp is a competitive plant that can beat out other weeds attempting to grow, so we could produce vast acreages of industrial hemp without the need for pesticides, herbicides, or crop dusting. Industrial

The Many Uses of Hemp

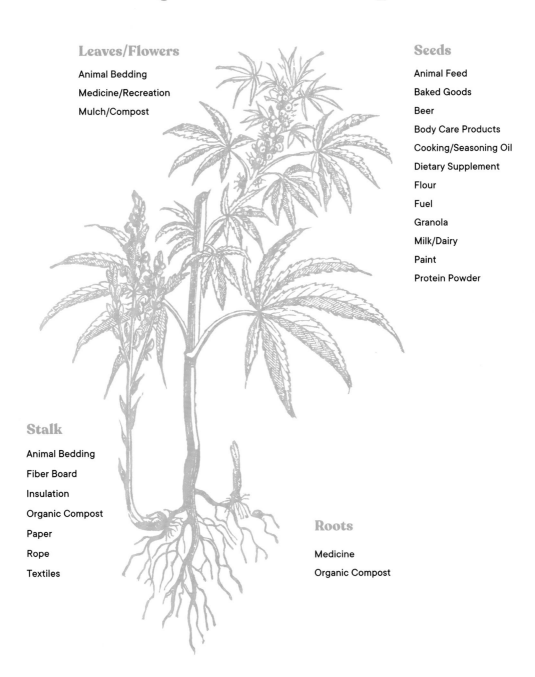

Leaves/Flowers

Animal Bedding

Medicine/Recreation

Mulch/Compost

Seeds

Animal Feed

Baked Goods

Beer

Body Care Products

Cooking/Seasoning Oil

Dietary Supplement

Flour

Fuel

Granola

Milk/Dairy

Paint

Protein Powder

Stalk

Animal Bedding

Fiber Board

Insulation

Organic Compost

Paper

Rope

Textiles

Roots

Medicine

Organic Compost

hemp has a large taproot capable of penetrating deep into the soil to pick up the required water and nutrients for plant development. This means hemp recovers nutrients that might otherwise be leached below the root zone and enter the groundwater. In addition, its deep roots open up the soil and enhance its tilth for future crops. Hemp also pulls carbon out of the earth and the air, more so than other crops.

Do we really need to keep going?!

Thankfully we're in the throes of a hemp renaissance. The US government is beginning to understand that hemp is a vital component to a sustainable nation. Earlier in this book, we discussed the rocky history of hemp and the many challenges it has faced. Big business, capitalist interests, and socioeconomic politics are opponents that rarely lose, but for once hemp has the support of both sides of the aisle. Now it's up to us, the caretakers of this planet. We are the future of hemp and, armed with the knowledge—and versatile recipes!—such as this book offers, we can begin to educate and build awareness about the power of hemp.

Let's take a look at how we incorporate our favorite hemp extract into our daily lives and actively participate in this hemp celebration.

Incorporating CBD

THE IMPORTANCE OF DAILY RITUALS

Good habits are the foundation of wellness. The reality is that even the best products are not overnight miracles; it's up to us to adapt our lifestyles to reach our ideal state of happiness. Our thoughtful and deliberate choices—to sign up for a yoga class, research and try CBD, buy organic bananas, or set aside ten extra minutes for self-care—are all based on the intention to live a stronger, healthier lifestyle. With intention, you can eventually turn those individual conscious decisions into rituals. Those rituals are what connect us to wellness and support us throughout our waking and sleeping hours.

We get it: it's not easy to form good habits. Especially if you need to lose the bad ones first. When we set our intention to be less stressed and sedentary (after years of staring at a computer screen all day), we started with two evening walks a week and sought CBD as an alternative to alcohol and other stress relievers. The first few walks were actually difficult—not so much in the physical sense but in forcing ourselves to turn off the television, get off the couch, and get moving. Believe it or not, after hours at work, it actually felt like *more* work just to put on tennis shoes.

By comparison, incorporating CBD felt easier in the beginning. The first few weeks we used it, we definitely felt a difference and were very optimistic about finding a healthier way to de-stress. The tricky part was remembering to dose every day. In fact, it took us months after our first try to remember to take a dose each morning and night. We weren't the experts we are now, and we didn't think of CBD as a part of our routine in the same way as brushing our teeth or drinking water. We only remembered to take it when we were already stressed. Over time, we found that leaving a bottle by the coffee maker and in the bathroom cabinet provided simple reminders to take our CBD when it really mattered. Today, we start and end each day with a dose of CBD oil and use it to supplement everything from an extra workout to a night of packing customer orders. It has allowed us to realize how important rituals are in maintaining the lifestyle we aspire to lead.

Sometimes treating yourself to a material object can inspire or motivate you to form better habits. Here are a few key items that have served as gentle reminders to make more conscious decisions or have complemented our CBD applications in beauty, fitness, or relaxation. While some products on the market turn out to be short-lived trends (fidget spinners, anyone?), these have continued to play a regular role in our own rituals and are some of the most treasured items in our home.

BINCHOTAN CHARCOAL STICKS: Filter and purify your water and enjoy the soft taste.

DIFFUSER: Use aromatherapy to improve your mood and get a better night's sleep.

DRY BRUSH: Gently exfoliate and detoxify your skin while encouraging blood circulation and lymphatic drainage.

FOAM ROLLER: Try it for increasing blood flow and oxygen to your muscles to reduce pain and improve flexibility.

FRUIT BOWL: Believe it or not, apples, tomatoes, peaches, and berries don't belong in the refrigerator. Keeping a bowl of fruit on the counter will remind you to reach for healthy snacks.

GLASS PITCHER: Stop giving plastic a second chance. He'll never change.

GUA SHA: Use this stone tool to firm your facial muscles and smooth the skin by promoting tissue drainage.

PALO SANTO STICKS: Burn these to cast out bad energy and invite creativity. The warm scent of the "holy wood" is divine.

SILK PILLOWCASES: Sleep on silk—it won't draw the moisture from your face into the fabric, plus it keeps sleep creases and bedhead at bay.

WINDOW PRISM: Hang one where you get the most natural light, and your new favorite time of day will be "rainbow o'clock" (as we like to call it), when the sun shines and refracts through the prism.

WIRELESS HEADPHONES: Don't let a cord keep you from bustin' a move.

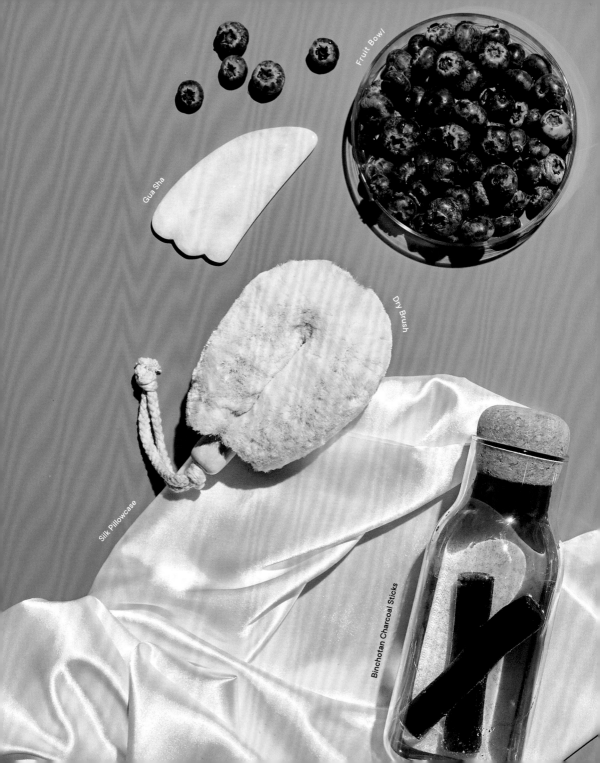

Fruit Bowl

Gua Sha

Dry Brush

Silk Pillowcase

Binchotan Charcoal Sticks

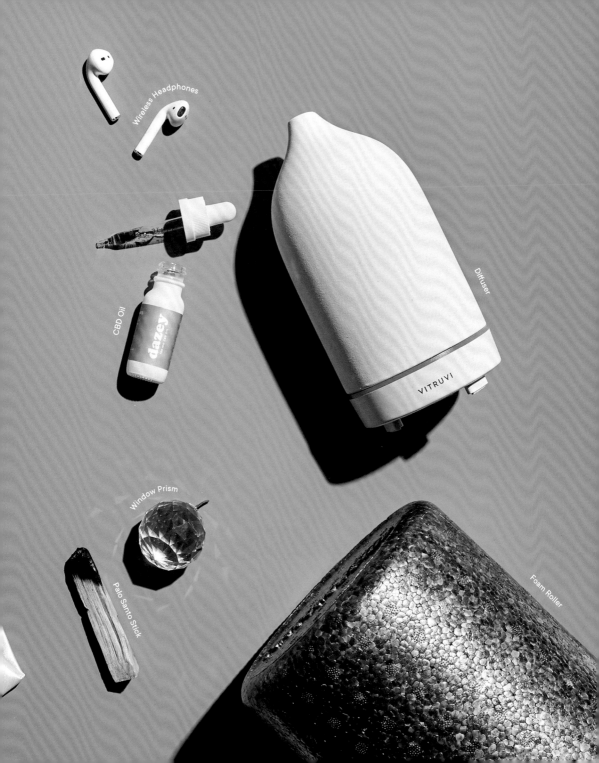

Wireless Headphones

Diffuser

CBD Oil

dazey

VITRUVI

Window Prism

Foam Roller

Palo Santo Stick

While everybody responds to CBD differently, there's no arguing that CBD could replace Windex as a personal cure-all in a modern remake of *My Big Fat Greek Wedding*. CBD's multipurpose application makes it incredibly easy to use in myriad recipes and situations. We initially turned to CBD for stress management, but now we use it to get glowing before date night, calm our nerves before a presentation, settle our stomachs when flying, or sleep through the night. No matter what life throws at you, there's a CBD recipe for that.

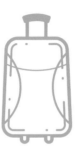

Leaving on a Jet Plane

- Cardamom Latte (page 58)
- Half-Baked Energy Bars (page 62)
- Ginger Chews (page 73)
- Caffeinated Eye Cream (page 114)
- Keep Swimming Stress Spray (page 118)

Self-Care Sunday

- Swedish Glögg (page 86)
- Strawberry Detoxifying Mask (page 109)
- Flower Power Tub Tea (page 126)
- Leg & Booty Mask (page 129)
- Crystal-Charged Body Oil (page 138)

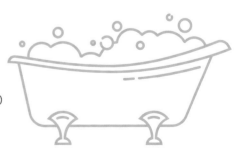

Date Night

- Moscow Mule (page 85)
- Manuka & Mint Lip Scrub (page 115)
- Personal Lubricant (page 134)
- Illuminating Body Butter (page 140)
- Baby Got Beard Oil (page 155)

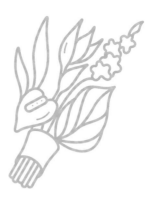

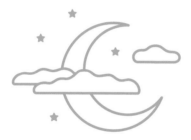

Sweet Dreams

- Midnight Moon Milk (page 81)
- Overnight Lip Mask (page 117)
- Keep Calm Stress Spray (page 118)
- Blemish Buster (page 120)
- Dry Scalp Elixir (page 151)

New Workout Class

- Blender Breakfasts (page 61)
- Old-Fashioned Fruit Rolls (page 71)
- Botanical Face Scrub (page 103)
- Grapefruit Cleansing Oil (page 104)
- Warming Muscle Rub (page 143)

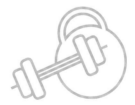

HOW TO USE THIS BOOK

You've made it to the fun part! We've put together seventy-five CBD-infused recipes to help you incorporate CBD into just about every part of your life. Each recipe is dosed using a one-milliliter dropper, the standard unit of measurement for most CBD oil on the market. One full dropper equals one milliliter. However, depending on the strength of your CBD oil, the total milligram dosage may vary. For example, one milliliter of Dazey's Mild formula contains twenty-five milligrams of CBD, whereas one milliliter of the Regular formula contains fifty milligrams. Take note of the strength of your CBD oil and the total milligrams in a full dropper so you can most closely align your dosage to the recipe. For continuity, we used Dazey's Regular formula for each recipe, and we've included both the total dropper amount and the total milligrams in the ingredients list. Of course, you're welcome to adjust the strength of the recipe by using a more or less concentrated CBD. It's entirely up to you!

You'll also notice Key Benefits called out for each recipe. We've provided recipes designed to help you relax, recipes to energize you, and recipes for recovery if you are looking for pain relief or management. On top of that, the Glossary (page 167) and Directory (page 176) supply all the tools you need to CBD & Chill.

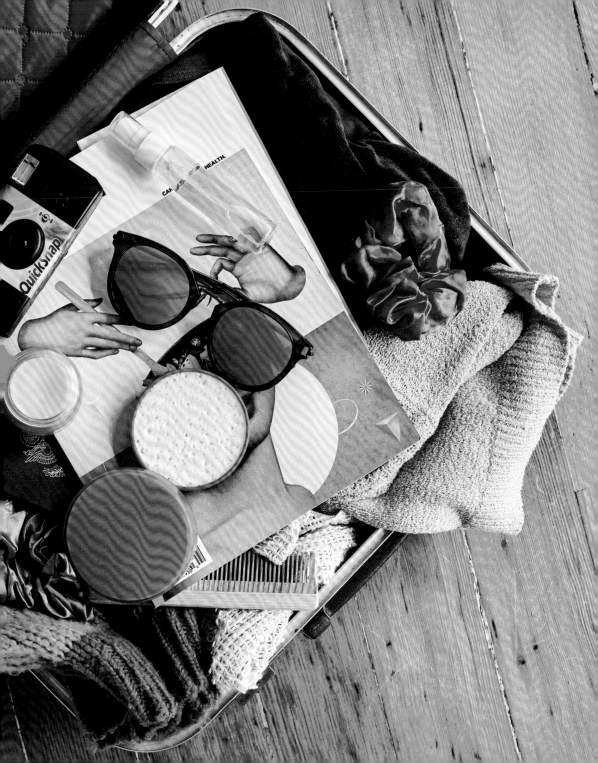

Part I

THE DAILY DOSE

Tasty Treats and Drinks for Everyday Wellness

COOKING WITH CBD

Cooking with cannabis can be a bit intimidating if you've never cooked with it before and are unsure of how it will react to heat, or how it might change the flavor of whatever you're making. Don't worry! You'll be a pro in no time.

Heat

Let's start with heat. While most of our recipes call for CBD to be added once the rest of the ingredients have been removed from heat, you may find variations or other online recipes that call for heat, so it's good to understand how temperature affects cannabis. Excessive heat *will* burn off cannabinoids and damage the naturally occurring terpenes of the oil. CBD begins to lose efficacy between 350 and 390 degrees F. Thankfully oven temperatures aren't food temperatures. Remember that Thanksgiving bird that roasted for hours at 350 degrees and came out with an internal temperature of only 165? As long as you stay away from the broil setting, you should be fine cooking cannabis in the oven.

Now when it comes to the stove top, you'll need to be a little more cautious. Stoves are measured by heat output (BTUs), not temperature, so it's not as easy to stay below 350 degrees. If you want to get super precise, you can use an infrared thermometer to measure the exact temperature of your pan while cooking. In general, however, we recommend staying in the medium-low range and avoiding anything higher than medium heat for an extended period. Whatever you do, *do not* let your oil begin to fry. At that point, you'll burn away all the beneficial compounds, and the excessive heat will turn your tasty oil into a bitter mess.

Butter and Oil

Fatty and oil-based ingredients bind well with cannabinoids and increase their bioavailability. That's why we blend our hemp extract with coconut oil. Not only is it perfect to cook with but it also tastes great! Keep your favorite fat or our Topping Oil (page 51) at the ready to take advantage of your hemp extract's full range of benefits.

STAPLE INFUSIONS

Let's start with a few tried-and-true infusions to kick things off. You'll want to keep these staples stocked in your cupboard or refrigerator for instant access to chill. Get yourself a few refillable jars because you'll go through these batches quickly. They're delicious and versatile, and you'll use them throughout this book. Master these staple infusions and you'll be ready to start whipping up your own CBD-infused recipes.

Each serving contains a small dose of CBD, perfect for complementing your daily dose and maintaining a clear head throughout the day. If you want these staples to serve as your only intake of CBD, feel free to bump up the milligrams to a dose that works for you.

Island Nut Butter

MAKES 4 CUPS

1½ cups dry-roasted, unsalted peanuts
1½ cups dry-roasted, unsalted almonds
1 cup dry-roasted, unsalted macadamia nuts
4 droppers CBD oil (200 milligrams)
Pinch of sea salt

TIPS:

- If you're on Team Crunchy, add 2 tablespoons flax or chia seeds for added texture.
- For a touch of sweetness, add 1 teaspoon ground cinnamon or vanilla extract.
- If you really want to feel like you're on a tropical getaway, add 2 tablespoons coconut flakes to complement the macadamia.

Nut butter is one of the most versatile staples. Slather it on toast, scoop it into a smoothie, or use it as a dip for veggies. Blended with a dose of CBD, just a tablespoon will give you a boost of energy and satisfy your cravings. After years of arguing over peanut versus almond butter, we started experimenting with different combinations and found that a blend of almond, peanut, and macadamia offers the creamiest flavor. Plus, the hint of macadamia will make you feel like you're on a Hawaiian vacation—even if just for a second.

1   In a food processor or high-speed blender, add the peanuts, almonds, and macadamia nuts. Let the machine run for a few minutes, scraping down the sides as needed, until the nuts release their oils and a creamy paste forms.

2   Add the CBD oil and salt and continue to process to the desired consistency. We like our nut butter on the thicker side, but you can add more coconut (or CBD) oil if you prefer a thinner consistency.

3   Scrape the nut butter into a mason jar with lid and store in the refrigerator. It will stay fresh for 3 to 4 months.

Local Wildflower Honey

MAKES 1 CUP

1 cup raw wildflower
   honey, preferably
   local
3 droppers CBD oil
   (150 milligrams)

Raw honey contains antioxidants and phytonutrients that pasteurized honey lacks. These nutrients have antibacterial and antimicrobial properties, giving raw honey a leg up when soothing sore throats and fighting infections. While the shelf life is shorter, the deliciously sweet and delicately floral taste will keep you coming back for another spoonful. Use this staple to sweeten cereal, fruit, or tea while microdosing your CBD! For this recipe, we chose a local honey sourced from wildflowers here in the Pacific Northwest. Consuming honey from your native region is said to reduce seasonal allergies by introducing a small amount of your local pollen into your system and building immunities against them. It's an easy way to stay connected with your surroundings and transition through the seasons.

1   In a double boiler, or in a heatproof bowl set over a pan of simmering water, heat the honey over low heat until it becomes thinner and easier to stir.

2   Add the CBD oil and stir for 1 to 2 minutes, being careful not to let the mixture simmer or boil. Do not exceed low heat.

3   Remove from the heat and pour the honey into a squeeze container or mason jar with lid. To enjoy, drizzle on foods or add to recipes. Each tablespoon contains about 9 milligrams CBD.

Topping Oil

MAKES 2 CUPS

1 (16.9-ounce) bottle
extra-virgin olive oil
(500 milliliters)
1 bottle or 15 milliliters
CBD oil (700
milligrams)

Olive oil is an ingredient you can use in just about anything—to make a salad dressing, drizzle on hummus, create a marinade, or whip up your favorite pasta dish. This CBD infusion is so versatile, you'll want to keep it on the counter for easy access. Every milliliter of this topping oil will give you a CBD dose of about 1.5 milligrams. Remember, this is not your everyday olive oil. This is your *special* olive oil.

1 Pour the entire bottle of olive oil into a small saucepan and place over low heat for 5 minutes.

2 Remove from the heat and stir in the CBD oil.

3 Pour the oil through a funnel back into the bottle. Do not use the oil in recipes that require cooking over high heat. Instead, use it as a topping or dressing to preserve the hemp extract's beneficial compounds.

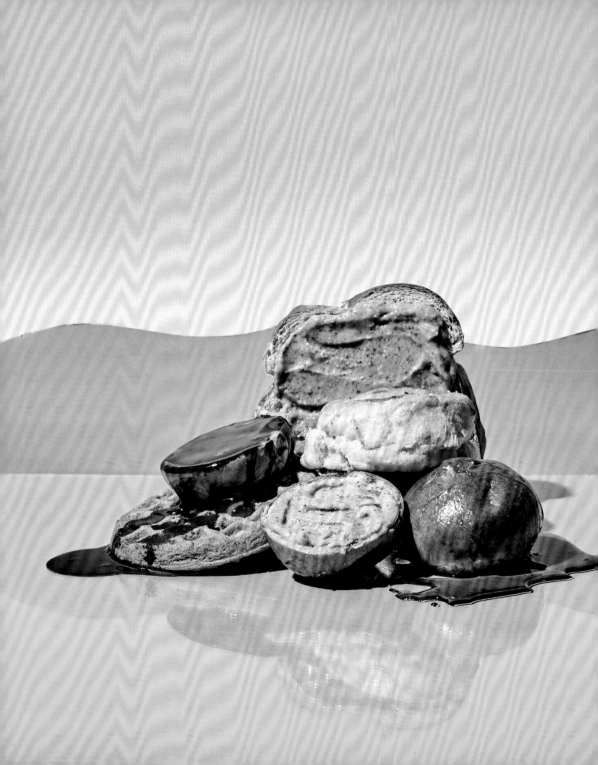

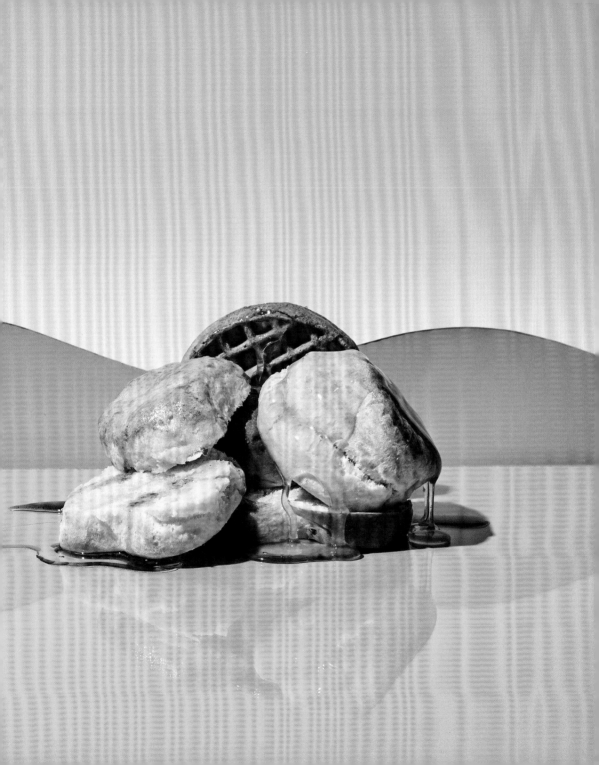

Espresso Maple Syrup

KEY BENEFITS:
Morning alertness,
caffeine moderation
(no jitters)

MAKES 1 CUP

1 cup Grade A amber-
color maple syrup
2 tablespoons organic
ground coffee or
espresso
2 droppers CBD oil
(100 milligrams)

Nothing says weekend quite like a cup of coffee and a stack of pancakes, waffles, or French toast topped with a drizzle of maple syrup. But we like to drink our coffee and eat it too, so we infused espresso directly into syrup for a rich, roasted flavor with a sweet finish that will awaken your senses.

1   Combine the maple syrup and ground coffee in a small saucepan. Bring to a simmer over medium heat and cook for 5 minutes to infuse the flavors. Remove from the heat.

2   Add the CBD oil and stir slowly for 1 minute.

3   Let steep for another 10 minutes and then pour the syrup through a strainer into a mason jar with lid or syrup dispenser. Serve warm or at room temperature. Each tablespoon contains about 6 milligrams CBD.

SURPRISING USES FOR MAPLE SYRUP:

- Substitute for the icing on cinnamon rolls.
- Drizzle on roasted pork or steak.
- Add to your favorite chocolate chip or oatmeal cookie recipe.
- Did someone say candied bacon?

Raw Cacao Sauce

MAKES ⅓ CUP

2 tablespoons coconut
oil
3 tablespoons raw
cacao powder
Pinch of sea salt
1 dropper CBD oil
(50 milligrams)

A good chocolate sauce is a sure way to satisfy your sweet tooth, no matter your dessert of choice. Hot chocolate, dipped fruit, ice cream topping: the possibilities are endless. Raw cacao is made from cold-pressing unroasted cacao beans, which maintains higher antioxidant levels than processed cocoa powder. It also contains phenethylamine, the scientific name for what is more commonly known as the "love chemical." It's a natural mood booster that stimulates the nervous system and triggers the release of endorphins. Needless to say, cacao and CBD are this century's greatest power couple. This recipe has a slightly higher potency than the other staples—about 16 milligrams per tablespoon—but we find that our chocolate cravings are often a by-product of high emotions, so why not satisfy and reset the mood?

1   Add the coconut oil to a small saucepan and heat it very gently at low heat until melted. Add the cacao powder and salt, and gently mix until dissolved.

2   Remove from the heat and add the CBD oil, stirring until smooth. Serve with your dessert of choice.

3   Store leftover sauce in a mason jar with lid in the refrigerator. If the sauce becomes too thick, place the jar in a bowl of warm water until it reaches drizzling consistency.

BREAKFAST

Breakfast: the most important meal of the day and the perfect time to jump-start your calm, cool, and collected self. These recipes cover everything you need to know about CBD and caffeine, as well as our favorite grab-and-go morning treats: smoothies and breakfast bars. Of course, you can also make a stack of pancakes drizzled with Espresso Maple Syrup (page 54) or spread Island Nut Butter (page 49) on toast when you're in a hurry. As long as CBD is in the mix, you'll be ready when someone throws a last-minute meeting on your calendar—and you know they will.

But First, Coffee

KEY BENEFITS:
Energy boost,
improved focus

MAKES 1 SERVING

What's better than opening your eyes after a restful night's sleep and smelling freshly ground coffee? Nothing, that's what. Caffeine, in general, actually synergizes really well with CBD. From relieving caffeine jitters to piggybacking on the improved focus that caffeine gives, CBD is a powerful ally for your cup of joe.

Have you ever felt overwhelmed by caffeine's heightened sense of alertness? Maybe you've had one cup too many and felt anxious or awkward? We've all been there. Coffee—and tea, shout-out to tea!—is delicious, and it's easy to overindulge. Thankfully there's a natural solution for those overcaffeinated situations: CBD! As caffeine sharpens your senses, CBD balances your mood and counteracts the adverse effects of a caffeine overdose.

When it comes to adding CBD to your coffee, the degree of effort you put into making your drink is totally up to you. Some mornings we simply drop our dose right on top of our brew. Other days, usually on weekends, we like to add CBD into our hemp milk as we steam it. Sometimes we create little CBD smiley faces in the foam. Have fun with it!

Cardamom Latte

2 teaspoons Local Wildflower Honey (page 50) (6 milligrams CBD)

2 shots espresso

½ cup almond milk

¼ dropper CBD oil (12 milligrams)

2 teaspoons ground cardamom, plus extra for garnish

1   Add the honey to the bottom of a mug or espresso glass. Whisk in the espresso.

2   In a separate cup, whisk the milk, CBD oil, and cardamom and then froth and heat the milk.

3   Top the espresso with the frothed milk and sprinkle with more cardamom before serving.

Cherry Espresso Soda

1 cup seltzer water or club soda

¼ dropper CBD oil (12 milligrams)

2 shots espresso

1 vanilla bean or 1 teaspoon vanilla extract

1 to 2 maraschino cherries

1   Fill a tall glass with ice. Pour in the seltzer and CBD.

2   Slowly add the espresso—it's going to be fizzy!—and garnish with the vanilla bean and cherries. Stir and enjoy.

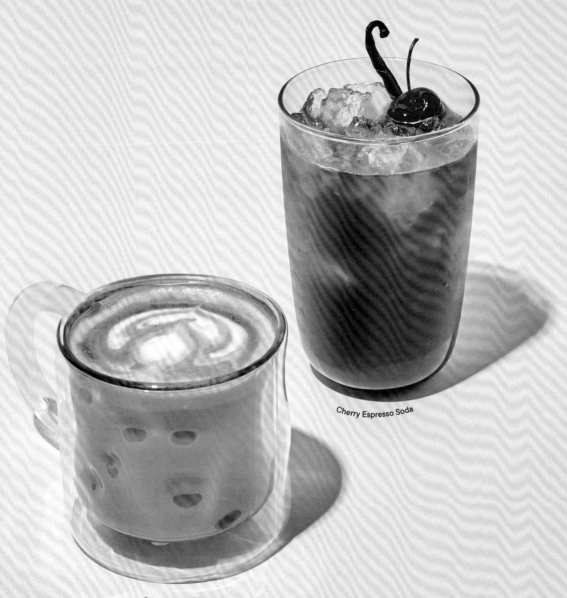

Cherry Espresso Soda

Cardamom Latte

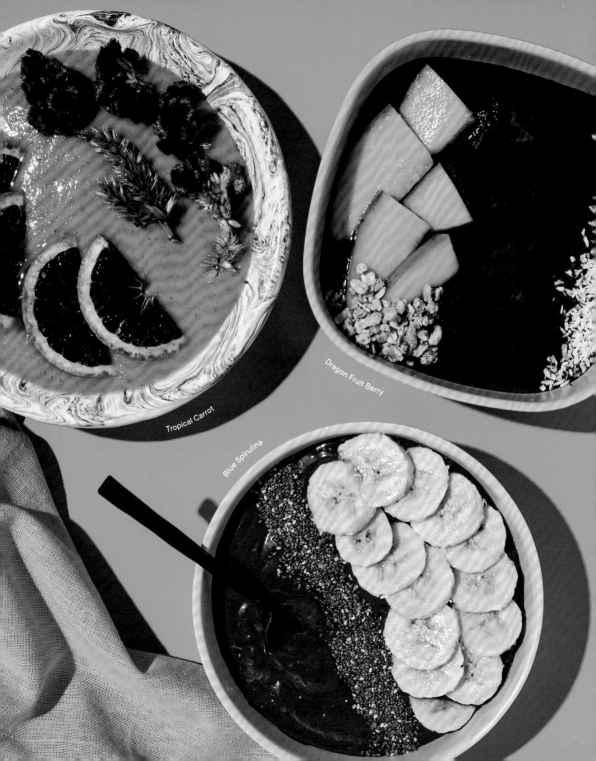

Tropical Carrot

Dragon Fruit Berry

Blue Spirulina

Blender Breakfasts

MAKES 1 SERVING

Its high sugar content makes fruit best in the morning, after our bodies have been shut down for the night and are ready to start up again. Blended with a dose of CBD, these smoothies include extraordinary ingredients that will counter your daily stress and give you a boost to start your day with clarity and energy.

Dragon Fruit Berry

2 (4-ounce) packets frozen
   dragon fruit
½ cup frozen mixed berries
1 medium banana, sliced

½ cup coconut milk
½ dropper CBD oil (25 milligrams)
Toppings: mango, granola,
   coconut flakes

Tropical Carrot

1 cup frozen mango
1 cup frozen pineapple
⅓ cup frozen strawberries
½ medium banana, sliced
1 small carrot, chopped

⅓ cup orange juice
⅓ cup pineapple juice
½ dropper CBD oil (25 milligrams)
Toppings: blood orange slices,
   edible flowers

Blue Spirulina

½ cup frozen acai berries
⅓ cup coconut cream
¼ cup vanilla almond milk
1 small orange
1 small ripe avocado
2 tablespoons almond butter

1 tablespoon spirulina powder
1 teaspoon honey
½ dropper CBD oil (25 milligrams)
Toppings: banana or kiwi slices,
   chia seeds, bee pollen

1   Combine all the ingredients for the desired variation in a blender and mix until smooth.

2   Transfer to a glass, to-go cup, or bowl, and sprinkle with granola or any of the suggested toppings.

Half-Baked Energy Bars

KEY BENEFITS:
Mood and
energy booster

MAKES 10 BARS

1 cup rolled oats
¼ cup flaxseeds
¼ cup hemp hearts
¼ cup coconut oil
1 cup pitted and
  chopped dates
½ cup chopped
  cashews
½ cup sliced almonds
¼ cup crushed banana
  chips
2 droppers CBD oil
  (100 milligrams)
Pinch of salt
½ cup unsweetened
  coconut flakes

Whether you're (literally) starved for time or trying to fend off a hunger attack, these half-baked bars are your secret weapon. Keep a few ready to go in your cupboard, desk, or purse. We eat them in between meetings, on road trips, after workouts, or even as late-night snacks. The blend of sweet and savory flavors makes them irresistible, and ten milligrams of CBD per bar allows you to maintain energy levels and mental clarity.

1   Preheat the oven to 350 degrees F. Line a rimmed baking sheet with parchment paper. Also line an 8-inch square glass baking dish with parchment paper.

2   In a large bowl, combine the oats, flaxseeds, hemp hearts, and coconut oil, and spread the mixture onto the prepared baking sheet. Bake for 10 minutes, stir to mix, then bake for another 5 to 10 minutes, or until golden brown. Allow to cool slightly.

3   Meanwhile, pulse the dates in a food processor or high-speed blender until they have a dough-like consistency. Add the cashews, almonds, banana chips, CBD oil, and salt. Pulse briefly to chop.

4   In a large bowl, combine the date mixture and the baked oats and mix well. Scoop the mixture into the prepared baking dish and press firmly to smooth and level it. Sprinkle coconut flakes on top and cover with plastic wrap. Place in the freezer for at least 1 hour before dividing into 10 bars. Store the bars in the refrigerator for 3 to 4 days or in the freezer for up to 1 month. It's also very possible that you'll eat them all in one day. No shame. They're freakin' delicious.

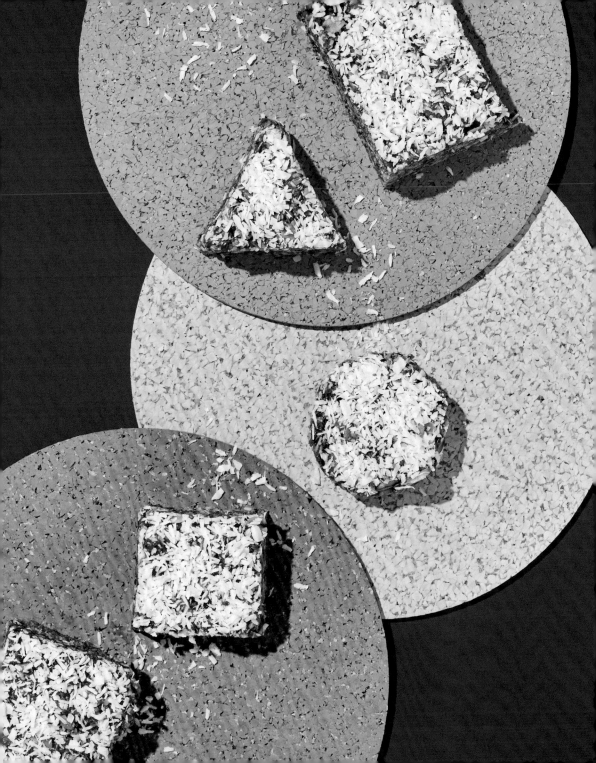

SNACKS

If there's one thing we always fall victim to, it's snack attacks. They always find us when we're the least prepared, and the only saving grace is a vending machine packed full of candy and sodium-heavy options. Fast forward to an hour later when we're bloated and two days later when we're desperately making a batch of Blemish Buster (page 120) to zap that giant zit that appeared overnight in the middle of our foreheads. Making these simple snacks in advance is one of the easiest ways to stay healthy and supplement your energy and focus through a dose of CBD. These palate-pleasers pack just the right punch to satisfy any craving.

Golden Beet Chips

MAKES 2 CUPS

6 large golden beets
(red works too),
scrubbed

½ teaspoon sea salt,
plus more for
sprinkling

2 tablespoons Topping
Oil (page 51) or
regular olive oil

1 teaspoon paprika

1 teaspoon ground
turmeric

½ dropper CBD oil
(25 milligrams)

1 lime wedge

Mmmm, chips. Chips are the go-to snack for binging the latest Netflix series, sure, but they're also guaranteed to fill you with feelings of regret and guilt. But no more! Now you can whip up some chips you can feel great about eating because these crunchy snacks are actually made of beets! By themselves, beets are packed full of fiber and vitamin C, but brushed with turmeric, CBD, and a dash of lime, they take superfood to the next level. Throw a batch in the oven at night and enjoy them the next day on their own or served alongside hummus, yogurt dip, cheese dip, guacamole, tzatziki . . . You get the idea.

1   Preheat the oven to 375 degrees F. Line a rimmed baking sheet with parchment paper.

2   With a sharp knife or a mandoline, thinly slice the beets, keeping them consistent in width. Lay them flat on the prepared baking sheet and sprinkle with salt. Let them sit for 10 minutes to "sweat" and then blot off the moisture. This will ensure they get extra crispy in the oven.

3   In a large bowl, toss the beets with the oil, paprika, turmeric, and ½ teaspoon salt. Return them to the baking sheet and bake in a single layer for 15 to 20 minutes, or until crispy and brown around the edges.

4   Return the beets to the bowl, add the CBD oil, and squeeze the juice from the lime wedge. Toss and lay flat again on the baking sheet until cool. Enjoy within 2 days for the best crunch!

Maple-Glazed Trail Mix

KEY BENEFITS:
On-the-go
energy

MAKES 3 CUPS

1 cup raw cashews

1 cup raw almonds

½ cup raw pecans

½ cup raw pumpkin
seeds

⅓ cup pure maple
syrup (our Espresso
Maple Syrup
on page 54 is a
delicious option for a
larger dose of CBD!)

1 tablespoon ground
cinnamon

1 teaspoon sea salt

4 droppers CBD oil
(200 milligrams)

A handful of this mix and you're ready for just about anything. Feel free to add in any other favorites like cacao nibs, dried cranberries, or mini marshmallows.

1   Preheat the oven to 350 degrees F. Line a rimmed baking sheet with parchment paper.

2   In a large bowl, combine all the ingredients, but reserve ½ dropper CBD oil. Transfer the mixture to the prepared baking sheet and bake for 10 minutes. Let cool completely and return to the bowl.

3   Toss the trail mix with the remaining ½ dropper CBD oil, along with any other favorite ingredients. Store in an airtight container at room temperature for up to 1 week.

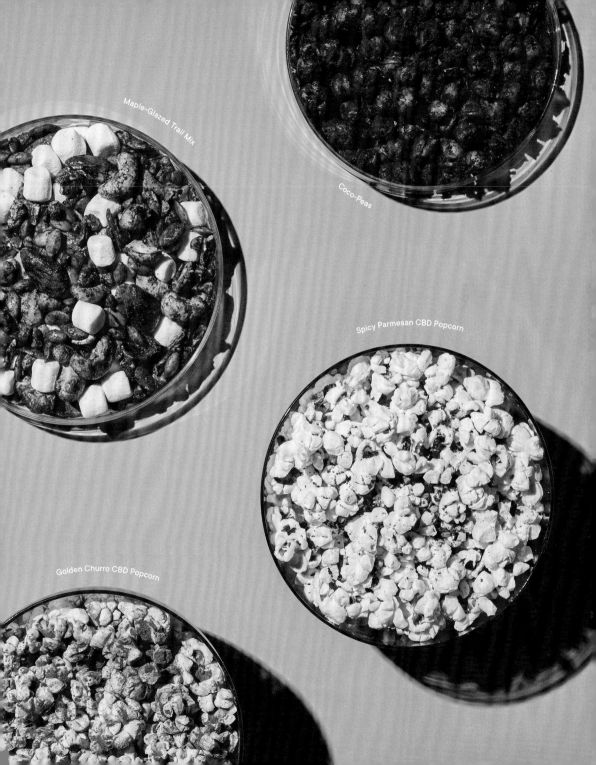

Maple-Glazed Trail Mix

Coco-Peas

Spicy Parmesan CBD Popcorn

Golden Churro CBD Popcorn

Sweet & Savory
CBD Popcorn

MAKES 4½ CUPS

Popcorn is a fantastic and healthy treat if you can manage to avoid an overload of butter, which is hard because . . . butter. Follow our instructions to air pop without any fancy equipment and then get creative with flavors. Go sweet or savory!

Spicy Parmesan

3 tablespoons popcorn kernels

2 droppers CBD oil
(100 milligrams)

3 tablespoons grated Parmesan cheese

¼ teaspoon paprika

¼ teaspoon red pepper flakes (optional, if you like it extra spicy)

¼ teaspoon sea salt

3 to 4 drops of your favorite hot sauce

TIP:

The fresher the kernels, the more water they contain inside their shells. When heated, the moisture trapped within creates the pressure that brings about the pop!

Golden Churro

3 tablespoons popcorn kernels

2 droppers CBD oil
(100 milligrams)

¼ cup coconut sugar

1 teaspoon ground cinnamon

½ teaspoon vanilla extract

Pinch of sea salt

1   To prepare the popcorn, preheat a 2-quart nonstick saucepan with a lid over medium heat for 5 minutes. Pour in the popcorn kernels and cover immediately.

2   Gently shake the pan every few seconds until the kernels start to pop, usually 1 to 2 minutes. Once 3 to 4 seconds elapse between pops, remove the pan from the heat. Pour the popcorn into a large bowl.

3   To prepare one of the seasoning blends, in a small bowl, combine all the ingredients. Add to the popcorn and mix well.

Coco-Peas

MAKES 2 CUPS

1 (15.5-ounce) can chickpeas (about 2 cups), rinsed, drained, and patted dry

2 tablespoons cocoa powder

2 tablespoons coconut or cane sugar

1 tablespoon coconut oil

½ teaspoon ground nutmeg

½ teaspoon sea salt

1 dropper CBD oil (50 milligrams)

Chickpeas (yes, also known as garbanzo beans) make a great snack because they're high in protein and fiber, which helps you feel a sense of fullness while aiding digestion. They also contain a range of vitamins and minerals, including iron, phosphate, calcium, potassium, magnesium, zinc, vitamins K and C, and choline. What's choline, you ask? It's an essential nutrient that plays a vital role in maintaining the structure of cellular membranes. It also supports nerve impulses throughout the body, making it a key player for reducing inflammation and aiding muscle movement. Paired with CBD and the rich flavor of cocoa powder, each tiny chickpea is a real powerhouse that perfectly satisfies both your sweet and savory cravings.

1 Preheat the oven to 450 degrees F. Line a rimmed baking sheet with parchment paper.

2 In a large bowl, toss the chickpeas with the cocoa powder, sugar, coconut oil, nutmeg, and salt. Pour the chickpeas onto the prepared baking sheet and bake for 20 minutes. Remove from the oven and return to the bowl.

3 Add the CBD oil and toss, then return the chickpeas to the baking sheet to cool. Enjoy fresh from the pan or store in a glass container in the refrigerator for up to 3 days.

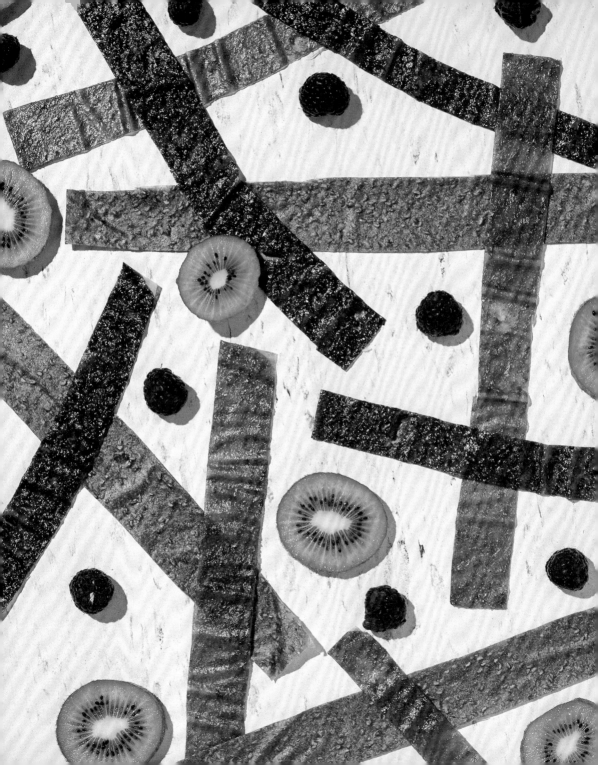

Old-Fashioned Fruit Rolls

KEY BENEFITS:
Vitamin-packed
energy booster

MAKES 8 ROLL-UPS

2 to 3 cups fruit (our
favorite combos are
listed at right)
3 tablespoons Local
Wildflower Honey
(page 50; 27
milligrams CBD)
2 tablespoons freshly
squeezed lemon
juice

This recipe is a throwback to elementary school, where we'd trade our entire lunch to the cool kids for a Fruit Roll-Up. Bonus points for the ones that gave you tongue tattoos. We like to think these rolls are just as fun, but they're a much healthier version without corn syrup or excess sugar. Don't be surprised if friends and strangers ask you to share or enter into modern-day trade negotiations.

Peach Raspberry

2 cups sliced peaches
½ cup raspberries

Strawberry Kiwi

2 cups whole strawberries
1 cup peeled kiwi

Pineapple Mango

2 cups sliced pineapple
1 cup sliced mango
1 teaspoon orange zest
Sprinkle of chili powder (for fans of
the mango carts in Los Angeles)

1 Preheat the oven to 140 degrees F (or as low as your oven will go). Line a rimmed baking sheet with parchment paper or a silicone baking mat.

2 Put the desired fruit in a blender or food processor and mix until smooth. Add the honey and lemon juice and pulse to combine.

3 Pour the mixture evenly onto the prepared baking sheet and spread it out to a thickness of ⅛ to ¼ inch. Bake for 3 to 5 hours, checking every 30 minutes after 3 hours, until the middle is no longer sticky to the touch. Remove from the oven and allow to cool completely.

4 Use clean scissors to cut the fruit roll into 1-inch strips. For a touch of nostalgia, cut parchment paper to match and roll them up. Keep refrigerated in an airtight container for up to 1 week.

DESSERTS & DRINKS

Perfect for large parties or a party of one, these dessert recipes will satisfy anyone with a sweet tooth and serve up a perfectly portioned dose of CBD. Whether you want to dish up the *chillest* desserts to friends, relax and savor the evening, or simply get ready for bed, these are the recipes we share the most often with friends and customers. We also show you how to incorporate CBD into your favorite alcoholic bevvies, or into mocktails that are refreshing for people of all ages.

Ginger Chews

MAKES 30 CHEWS

1 cup water
¾ cup fresh ginger,
    peeled and sliced
    into pieces ⅛ to
    ¼ inch thick
1¼ cups granulated
    sugar, divided
2 droppers CBD oil
    (100 milligrams)
Coarse sea salt

You're not alone if anxiety often makes you feel sick to your stomach. The anticipation of public speaking or trying something new can overwhelm your entire body. With a savory sweetness and the spice of ginger, these little guys will calm nervousness and nausea no matter what you're up against.

1   Place a cooling rack above parchment paper, preferably inside a dish or sheet pan, and set aside.

2   In a small saucepan over medium-high heat, combine the water and ginger. Cover and cook for about 30 minutes, or until the ginger is slightly tender.

3   Strain the ginger, reserving the water from the saucepan, then return the ginger to the saucepan with ¼ cup of the ginger water and 1 cup of the sugar.

4   Over medium heat, stir frequently until the water turns to a thick, syrup-like consistency and has mostly evaporated, about 20 minutes. The syrupy consistency is the key to this recipe. Remove from the heat, strain, and toss with the CBD oil.

5   Place the ginger pieces on the cooling rack and let cool completely.

6   Once cooled, toss the pieces with the remaining ¼ cup sugar and sea salt to taste. Return to the rack and let dry for at least a few hours, preferably overnight. Transfer to an airtight container and store in the refrigerator for up to 2 weeks.

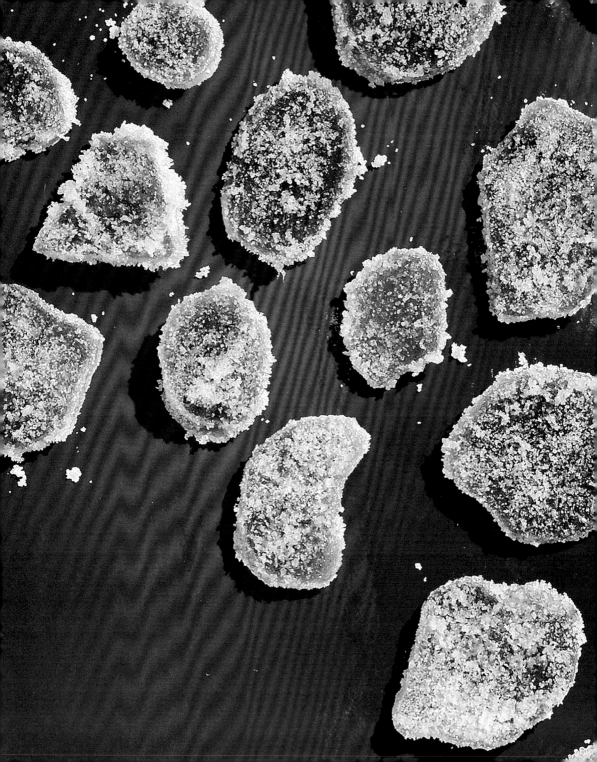

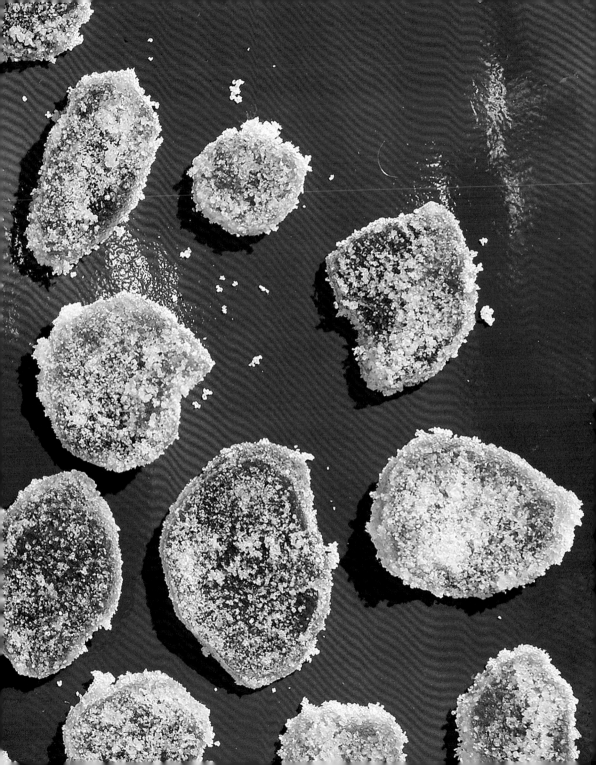

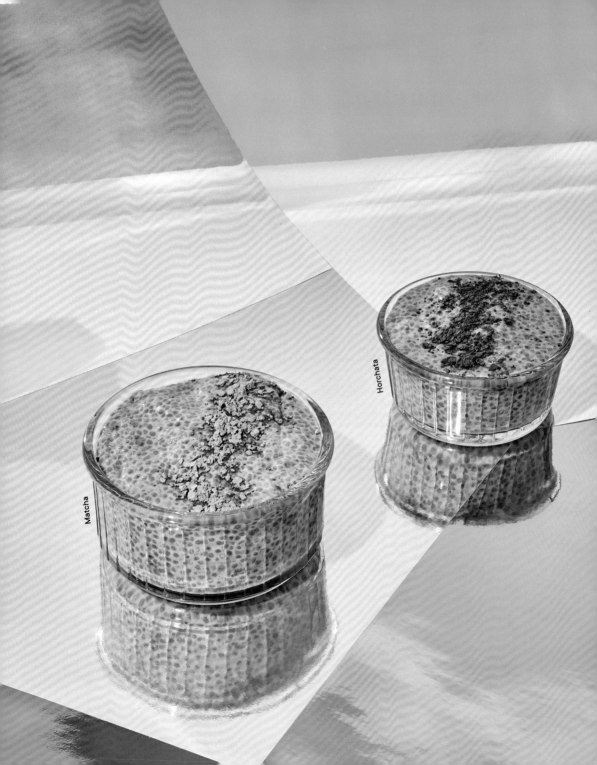

Matcha

Horchata

Chia Pudding

KEY BENEFITS:
Full of fiber

MAKES 2 CUPS

Overnight oats are so last year. Enter chia pudding: a deliciously easy dish that will keep you satisfied for hours. Chia seeds can hold ten times their weight in liquid and transform into *boba*-like bubble balls that are just as fun to eat as they are nutritious. Plus, the superfood pairs well with CBD, adding omega-3 fatty acids, fiber, protein, and amino acids to CBD's nutritional profile. We tend to revisit Chia Pudding over and over again, adding the flavors of matcha and horchata to make a tasty treat. Try experimenting with your own favorite flavors or toppings. Our rule of thumb is two tablespoons of chia seeds for every half cup of milk. If you have a sweet tooth, feel free to sweeten to taste.

Matcha

½ cup dairy-free milk (we prefer hemp or oat)
½ cup coconut milk
¼ cup chia seeds
1 teaspoon matcha powder

½ teaspoon vanilla extract
2 tablespoons Local Wildflower Honey (page 50; 18 milligrams CBD) or Espresso Maple Syrup (page 54; 12 milligrams CBD)

Horchata

½ cup dairy-free milk
½ cup coconut milk
¼ cup chia seeds
2 teaspoons cacao powder

2 tablespoons Local Wildflower Honey (page 50; 18 milligrams CBD)
1 teaspoon ground cinnamon

To prepare the pudding, combine all the ingredients for the desired variation in a medium bowl. Mix well to avoid clumping. Cover and refrigerate for at least 2 hours (overnight is best).

Nice Cream

MAKES 3 CUPS

Whether we're giving in to a sweet tooth or needing a treat to pair with our favorite romantic comedy, ice cream is usually a top contender. But dairy isn't everyone's friend. Our "nice creams" can be made with milk or a dairy-free alternative of your choice, and the flavor combinations are only limited by your imagination. And the best part is you don't need a fancy ice cream maker to dish up your own pint. You can even serve it with CBD toppings like our Raw Cacao Sauce (page 55) or Local Wildflower Honey (page 50).

Summer Strawberry

3 cups frozen strawberries,
   coarsely chopped
2 cups coconut milk

⅓ cup Local Wildflower Honey
   (page 50; 50 milligrams CBD)

CB&A (Chocolate, Banana & Avocado)

2 bananas, sliced
1 ripe avocado
1 cup coconut cream

1 cup oat milk
¼ cup Raw Cacao Sauce (page 55;
   25 milligrams CBD)

Salted Purple Potato

2 cups coconut milk
1½ cups purple sweet potatoes,
   peeled, steamed, and chopped
½ cup pure maple syrup

1 dropper CBD oil (50 milligrams)
2 teaspoons vanilla extract
1 teaspoon sea salt

To prepare the ice cream, combine all the ingredients for the desired variation in a blender and mix until smooth. Transfer to a bowl or loaf pan, cover tightly, and freeze for at least 3 hours before serving.

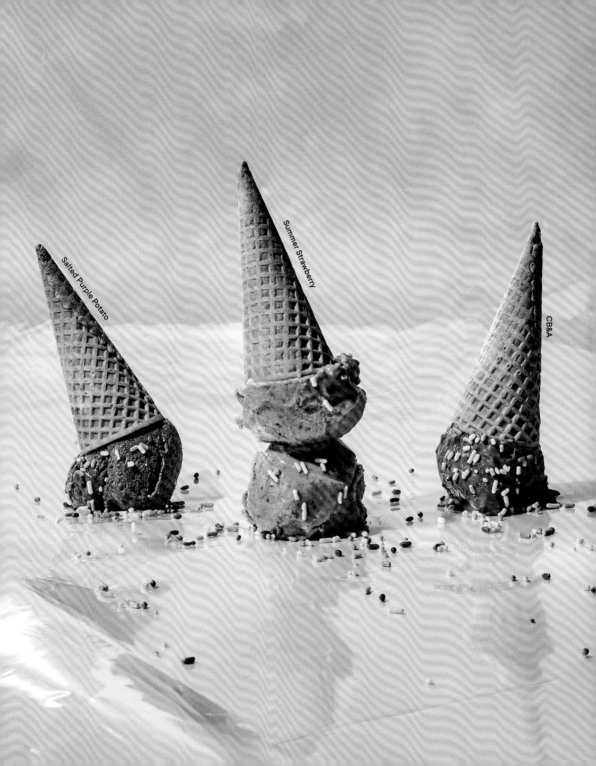

Salted Purple Potato

Summer Strawberry

CB&A

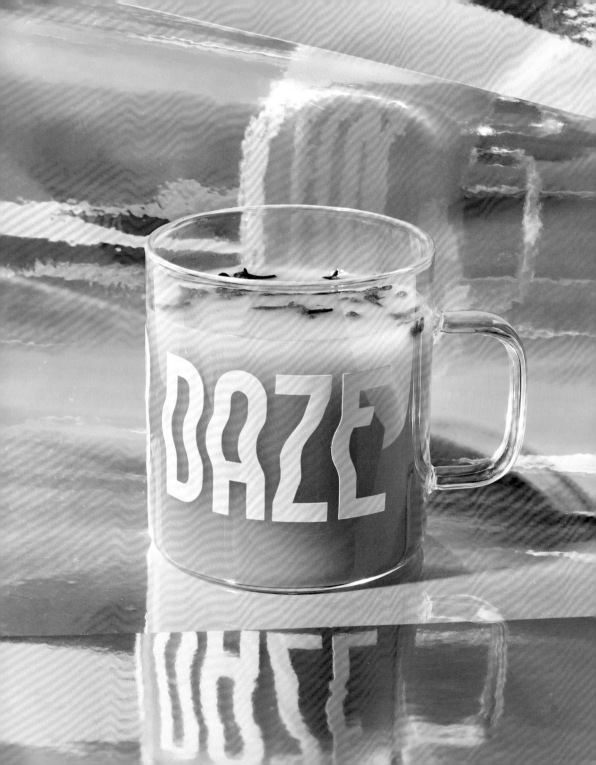

Midnight Moon Milk

MAKES 2 CUPS

2 cups dairy-free milk
    of choice
½ dropper CBD oil
    (25 milligrams)
2 teaspoons pure
    maple syrup
1 teaspoon
    ashwagandha root
    powder
½ teaspoon ground
    cinnamon, plus more
    for garnish
¼ dropper butterfly pea
    extract
Pinch of ground
    nutmeg
Pinch of ground
    cardamom
Whole cloves, for
    garnish

Ayurveda is one of the world's oldest healing systems, developed thousands of years ago in India. The "whole body" approach is centered on the belief that wellness depends on the balance of your mind, body, and spirit. An ancient tradition of Ayurveda, moon milk is considered a remedy for insomnia thanks to its blend of ashwagandha and spices in warm milk. We love the ritual of moon milk before bed, and the addition of CBD will combat sleeplessness and settle the mind even further. Our recipe gets its moody midnight color from butterfly pea extract, which we found while touring an herb farm on the island of Kauai. Butterfly pea is a traditional Ayurvedic ingredient to enhance memory and brain health, and it is recognized in more modern times for its ability to reduce stress and depression. As we sat among the growing flowers on Hawaii's "Garden Island," we couldn't resist the vibrancy of the extract's purple-and-blue hue. It's been our best souvenir to date.

In a small saucepan, heat the milk over medium heat until it starts to froth. Add in the CBD oil, maple syrup, ashwagandha, cinnamon, butterfly pea extract, nutmeg, and cardamom. Whisk until dissolved and pour into a glass or mug. Top with cloves and an extra dash of cinnamon.

Cocktail & Mocktail

Ready to get your drink *and* your chill on? Maybe you want to spike that mocktail with a little CBD? Let's cover a few known facts about CBD and alcohol before you start dosing that drink.

Both alcohol and CBD are known to relax and lower inhibitions, and these effects may compound when you mix the two. But there may also be benefits to combining. In a study published in *Psychopharmacology*, the combination of alcohol plus CBD resulted in significantly lower blood alcohol levels for participants compared to alcohol alone. However, few differences were observed between a group given alcohol alone and a group given alcohol plus CBD. The study concluded that neither compound will change how the other affects your motor or mental performance. In other words, whatever your usual state when drinking, be it happy or sad or somewhere in between, CBD will most likely not change that.

That said, there isn't much research on the topic, and it would be disingenuous to make scientific claims about combining alcohol and CBD. So, if you're planning to mix, be smart about it. Stay hyperconscious of your consumption levels, listen to your body, and take it slow. And of course, have fun!

Our favorite way to mix alcohol and CBD is to use ginger beer. Here in Seattle, Rachel's Ginger Beer creates the most delicious ginger brew you've ever tasted. From their original flavor to seasonal creations like pink guava or spicy pineapple, their straightforward recipe uses only lemons, ginger, cane sugar, and fresh water. They sell online and we highly recommend checking them out. Of course, your favorite grocery store ginger beer or home infusions will do the trick as well.

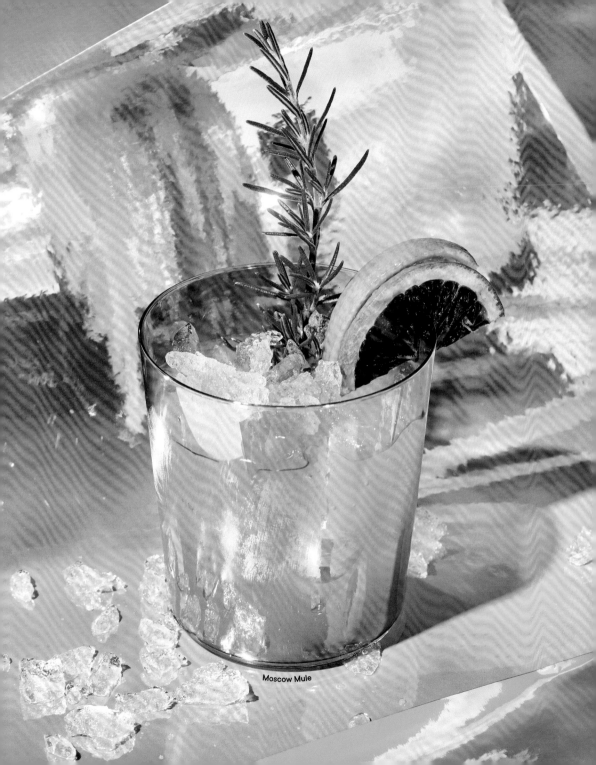

Moscow Mule

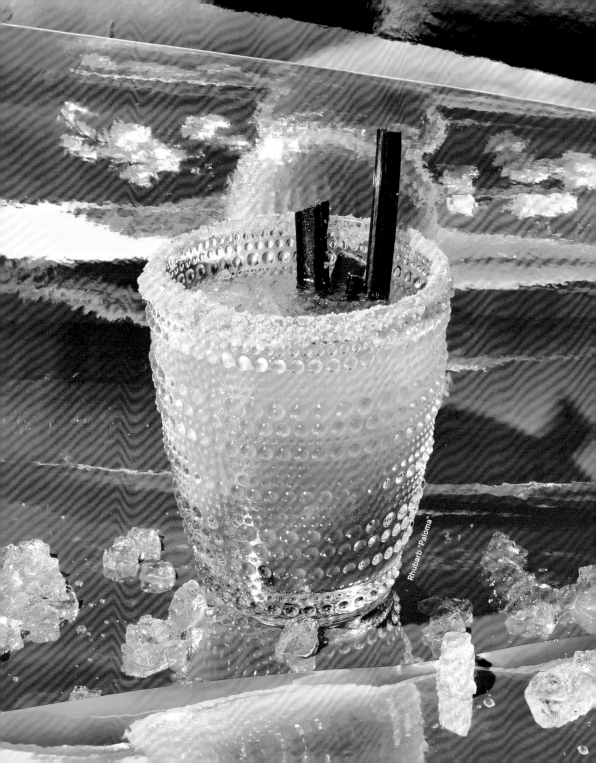

Rhubarb "Paloma"

Moscow Mule

¼ cup (2 ounces) vodka
1 tablespoon freshly squeezed
    lime juice

¼ dropper CBD oil (12 milligrams)
½ cup ginger beer
1 lime wedge, for garnish

Fill a copper mug or tall glass with ice. Add the vodka, lime juice, and CBD oil. Top with ginger beer and stir to combine. Garnish with a lime wedge.

TIP:

If you prefer a cocktail, add ¼ cup (2 ounces) tequila blanco.

Rhubarb "Paloma"

Pink Himalayan salt, for the rim
2 tablespoons Rhubarb Shrub,
    homemade (recipe follows) or
    store-bought
¼ cup freshly squeezed red or
    pink grapefruit juice

1 tablespoon freshly squeezed
    lime juice
¼ dropper CBD oil (12 milligrams)
¼ cup club soda
Ribbons of thinly shaved rhubarb
    and slices of lime or grapefruit,
    for garnish

1   Wet the rim of a tall glass with water and dip it onto a plate of Himalayan salt. Fill the glass with ice.

2   Add the rhubarb shrub, grapefruit and lime juices, and CBD oil, and then top with club soda. Weave the rhubarb ribbons and lime or grapefruit slices on a cocktail stick for garnish.

RHUBARB SHRUB (makes 2 cups)

| 2 cups water | 2 stalks rhubarb, chopped | 1 cup sugar |

1   In a medium saucepan, bring all the ingredients to a boil. Reduce the heat and let simmer for 10 minutes.

2   Remove from the heat and pour into a fine-mesh strainer or a colander lined with cheesecloth. Discard the solids and let cool. Store in the refrigerator for up to 6 months.

Swedish Glögg

MAKES 10 TO 12 SERVINGS

1 (750–milliliter) bottle
red wine
1½ cups vodka,
bourbon, or aquavit
1 tablespoon
cardamom seeds
½ tablespoon whole
cloves
2 twists of orange peel
1 cinnamon stick
2 tablespoons
blanched slivered
almonds
2 tablespoons raisins
2 droppers CBD oil
(100 milligrams)

Given Tori's heritage, it's surprising that there aren't more
Swedish recipes in this book. Glögg is a variation of mulled wine
and is well suited for CBD since it's enjoyed during the joyous
(and sometimes stressful) holiday season. Glögg is a traditional
Swedish alcoholic drink, a cross between mulled wine and a hot
toddy. It's sure to keep you warm and cozy, while a dose of CBD
will keep you merry and bright.

1   Combine the red wine, liquor of choice, cardamom, cloves, orange
    twists, and cinnamon stick in a large pot. Simmer for a minimum of
    1 hour.

2   Use a hand strainer to remove the cardamom seeds and cloves.

3   Remove from the heat and add the almonds, raisins, and CBD. Stir
    well to incorporate. Serve with a ladle.

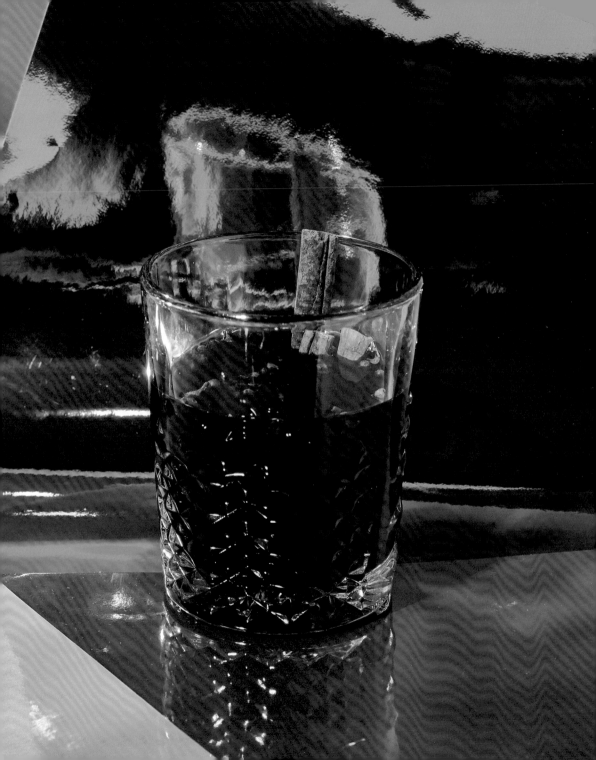

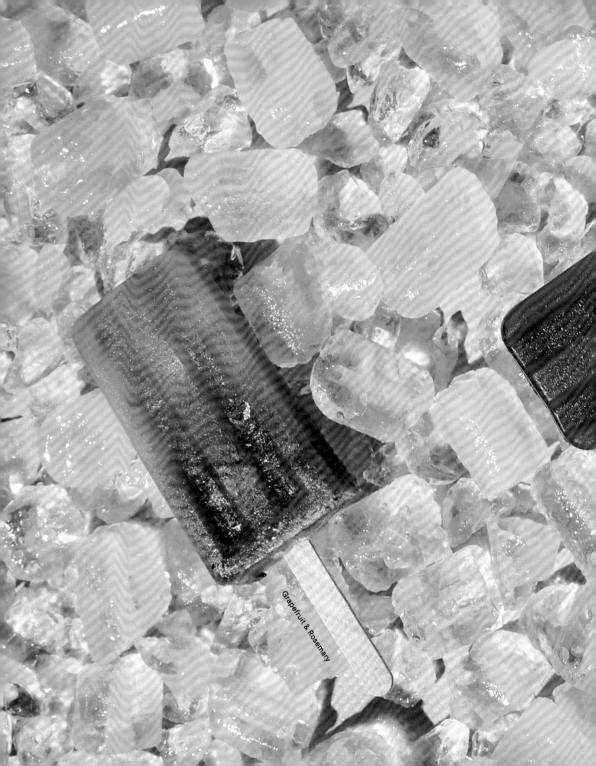

Grapefruit & Rosemary

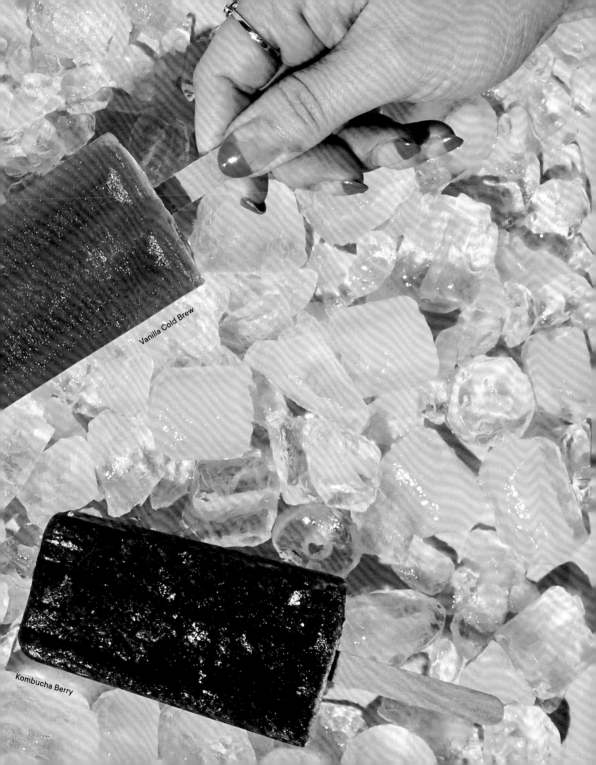

Vanilla Cold Brew

Kombucha Berry

Frozen Pops

MAKES 10 FROZEN POPS

If you want to be the most popular party host this summer, all you need are frozen pop molds and these recipes. They're the perfect treat to keep everyone chill—in more ways than one. For a more adult treat, try serving the pops upside down in a cup of prosecco or cold brew.

Vanilla Cold Brew

12 ounces unsweetened cold brew
3 ounces coconut milk

2 tablespoons Espresso Maple Syrup (page 54; 12 milligrams CBD)
1 teaspoon vanilla extract

Kombucha Berry

2 cups kombucha
1 cup strawberries, thawed if frozen

1 cup blueberries, thawed if frozen
½ dropper CBD oil (25 milligrams)

Grapefruit & Rosemary

2 cups chopped grapefruit, (membrane removed)
1½ cups club soda
½ cup sugar

2 teaspoons chopped fresh rosemary leaves
½ dropper CBD oil (25 milligrams)

1   Put all the ingredients for the desired variation in a blender or food processor and mix until smooth.

2   Pour the mixture into molds and insert wood sticks, if needed. Freeze for at least 6 hours.

3   Remove the pops from the molds. If necessary, run warm water over the molds to loosen the pops. Store flat in a gallon-size ziplock freezer bag for up to 6 months.

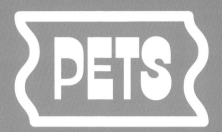

Humans aren't the only ones suffering from anxiety and bodily pain. Our four-legged friends can become anxious over loud noises or struggle to walk due to arthritis and stiff joints. The good news is that CBD can be just as helpful for dogs and cats as it is for us. Research on dogs has shown that CBD can reduce swelling and the frequency of seizures. For dogs and cats, we recommend up to five milligrams for every ten pounds of weight. Of course, you should consult with your veterinarian before administering CBD, especially for pets already on any medications.

Our own dog (pictured on the following pages) is an Australian Shepherd mix. As intelligent as she is, a single beeping noise sends her shivering into the closet. To keep her calm in stressful situations—travel, trips to the vet, facing the dreaded vacuum—we give her a dose of twenty-five milligrams of CBD oil about thirty minutes beforehand. Daily, we add a few drops (five milligrams) to her breakfast and dinner. We've seen noticeably lower levels in her anxiety in new situations, and improved flexibility and recovery time after hours of Frisbee. Even her fur seems healthier and shinier. Plus, she loves the taste! If you've ever tried to trick a dog into swallowing a pill hidden in cheese or peanut butter, you'll understand what a relief it is to have a medication your dog won't spit out. But if your dog is a picky eater or you want to provide a treat that is delicious and healthful, try our Pumpkin & PB Dog Treats or Banana Soft-Serve. They're winners with all the pups we know.

Pumpkin & PB Dog Treats

KEY BENEFITS: Settles the stomach, reduces anxiety

MAKES 24 TREATS

1 (15–ounce) can
    pumpkin puree
    (without additives)
¼ cup peanut butter
    (without xylitol and
    added sugar or salt)
¼ cup coconut oil
1 dropper CBD oil
    (50 milligrams)

No tricks required for this treat. Not only is this recipe easy (and cost effective!) to prep, but the simplicity also makes it a healthy alternative to mass-produced treats that may be using everything from corn gluten to meat or grain by-products, food dyes, or chemical preservatives as key ingredients. We've based this recipe on two of the natural ingredients our dog loves most: pumpkin and peanut butter. Pumpkin is an excellent source of fiber and is known to help ease stomach issues, while peanut butter is packed with protein, heart-healthy fats, and vitamins B and E. When combined with a microdose of CBD, these treats are our go-to for maintaining a happy and healthy doggo disposition.

1   In a medium saucepan, heat all the ingredients over low heat until liquefied into the consistency of a thick soup. You don't want to burn off the CBD, so keep the heat at or below medium-low.

2   Remove from the heat and pour the mixture into silicone ice cube trays. Freeze for at least 2 hours or until hardened.

3   Pop the treats out of the trays, place in ziplock bags, and store in the refrigerator for up to 2 weeks.

4   Serve 1 cube to your dog about 20 minutes before high-anxiety events, such as trips to the vet, car rides, or walks. Treats can also be given daily in lieu of directly administered oil, especially if your dog isn't feeling the taste of straight CBD. For larger dogs, increase the total CBD in this recipe from 50 milligrams—about 2 milligrams per treat— to 100 milligrams or 150 milligrams, depending on your dog's weight.

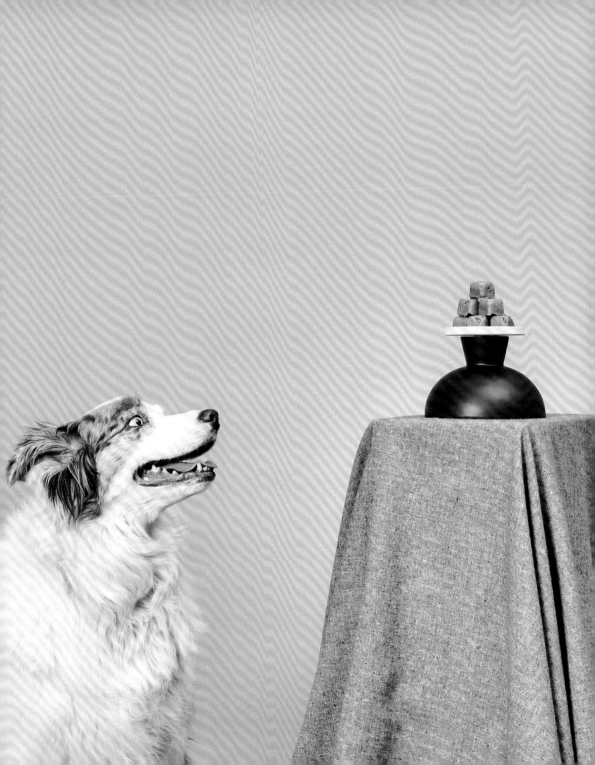

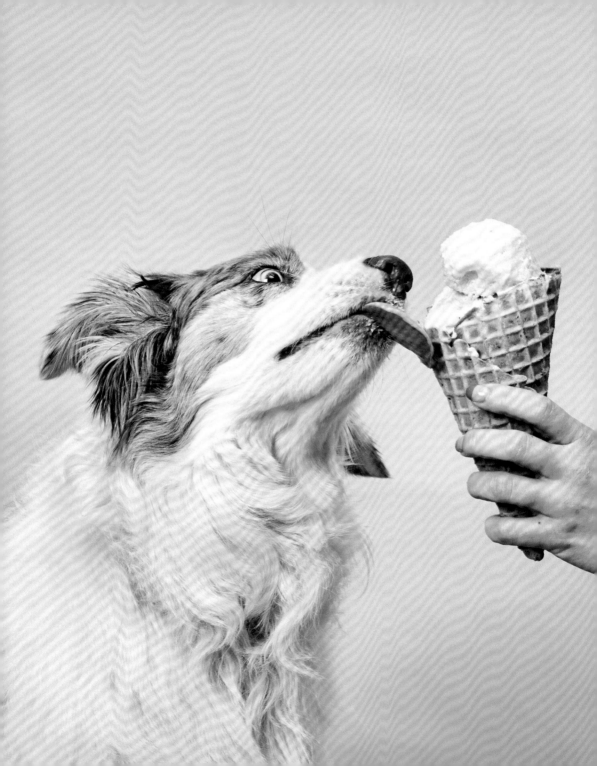

Banana Soft-Serve

KEY BENEFITS:
Cold-packed
potassium

MAKES 5 CUPS

24 ounces plain yogurt
1 cup sliced banana
½ cup coconut oil
½ dropper CBD oil
(25 milligrams)

Cue Gwen Stefani because this summer treat is B-A-N-A-N-A-S. If you have an energetic dog like ours, you're probably always looking for creative ways to keep them entertained. During warmer months, we found that an ice block was a great way to keep her cool and busy as she licked it down to the center. We rotate between frozen chicken broth, frozen cubes with treats inside, and this recipe. By far, the banana soft-serve is her favorite. She goes wild for the prebiotic- and potassium-packed banana flavor and usually spends the rest of the afternoon resting in the shade.

1   Put all the ingredients in a blender and mix until smooth.

2   Pour the mixture into a freezer-safe container or silicone ice cube trays. Treat your dog to a scoop or cube during warm summer days. Each cup contains about 5 milligrams CBD.

Part II

GO FOR THE GLOW

CBD Beauty, Skin Care, and Topical Remedies

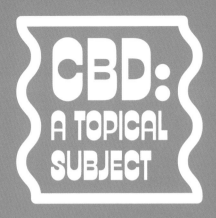

CBD has established itself as an internal remedy against anxiety, pain, and insomnia for many people. It's also an increasingly popular ingredient in beauty and skin care treatments as we learn more about how CBD interacts with and benefits our skin. There are two ways to use CBD topically: in higher concentrations for pain and in lower concentrations for skin health. In higher concentrations, usually two hundred milligrams and above, CBD is used to target specific areas of discomfort as it absorbs through the skin down to the muscle layer to help combat soreness and stiffness. In lower concentrations, CBD is popping up in products ranging from facial oil to shampoo for its anti-inflammatory properties and ability to regulate oil production. The tricky part is vetting those products and being careful not to succumb to deceptive marketing that likens hemp seed oil—often labeled *Cannabis sativa* seed oil and long available in health food stores— to real CBD oil, which is made from the entire hemp plant rather than just the seeds.

Incorporating quality CBD into products you make yourself is one of the easiest and most reliable ways to test different topical formulations. CBD is just one of the many botanical ingredients in the recipes that follow, where you'll discover many healing plants and fruits that complement hemp's ability to nourish, moisturize, and restore.

We recommend that you perform a patch test for any unfamiliar ingredients to help predict possible negative side effects. If any irritation occurs, find a substitute that works better for you. For all recipes, please use stainless-steel utensils and bowls whenever possible, sterilize with rubbing alcohol to prevent contamination, and store all products in a cool, dark place, unless otherwise noted. In the Directory on page 176, we've also listed our favorite websites for purchasing the ingredients, containers, and tools used in our topical recipes.

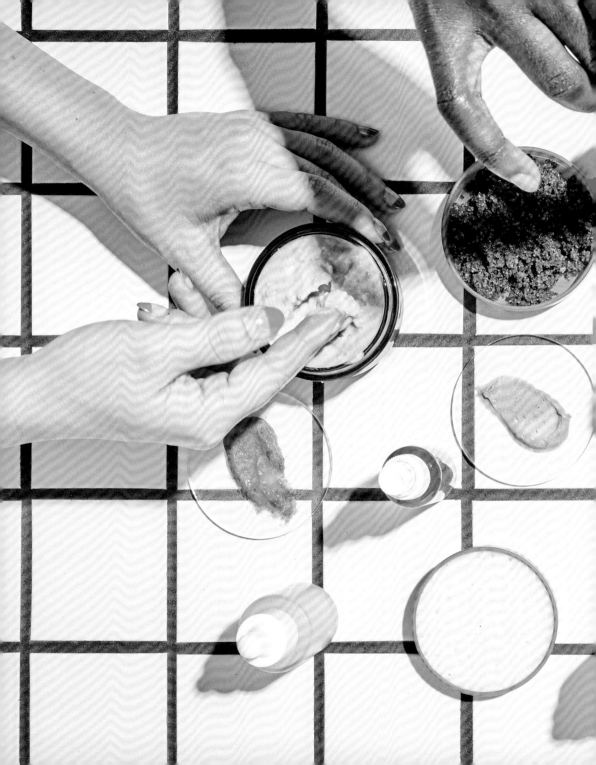

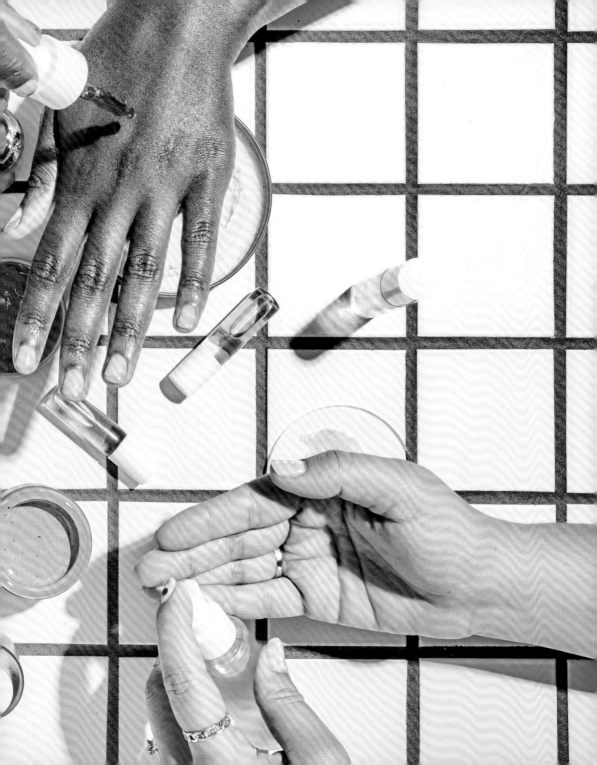

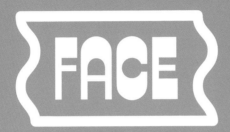

Shortly after launching our company, we added one hundred milligrams of CBD into one of our favorite facial oils to see if it would really make a difference. It was the middle of winter, and we were both struggling to keep our T-zone from drying out. It's no exaggeration when we say we saw dramatic differences within the first few days of use, and adding CBD was the only thing that had changed. Our skin was still soft in the morning and didn't feel desert-dry after a morning wash. Since then, we have continued to be impressed with CBD and have seen it help customers across the skin care spectrum. Whether your skin is acne-prone, oily, or irritated, you'll find formulations that harness CBD to revitalize the skin cells on your face and nurture problem areas. Even your lips will thank you!

Botanical Face Scrub

MAKES 2 OUNCES

3 tablespoons shea
    butter
5 milliliters rose hip oil
5 milliliters
    pomegranate seed
    oil
1 teaspoon spirulina
3½ ounces (100
    milliliters) organic
    cold-pressed aloe
    vera gel
1 tablespoon jojoba
    esters
2 droppers CBD oil
    (100 milligrams)

A regular exfoliating routine removes the barrier of dead skin cells from the top layer of your skin and allows other moisturizing products to penetrate more deeply and effectively. However, over-exfoliation can cause dryness and irritation, so most people should incorporate this gentle routine just twice a week. Our facial scrub avoids harsh agents like sulfates and alcohol and instead relies on the soothing properties of aloe and oils. Spirulina and CBD decrease inflammation and tone the skin alongside jojoba esters: tiny, solid forms of jojoba oil that are completely biodegradable.

1   In a double boiler, or in a heatproof bowl set over a pan of simmering water, melt the shea butter and then stir in the rose hip oil, pomegranate seed oil, and spirulina. Remove from the heat.

2   In a small bowl, combine the shea butter mixture with the aloe vera gel. Using an immersion blender or milk frother, slowly add the jojoba esters and CBD oil and mix until well blended. Pour the scrub into a 60-milliliter (2-ounce) container and let cool.

3   Apply an almond-size amount to your face in a circular motion to buff the skin. Rinse with warm water.

Grapefruit Cleansing Oil

MAKES 2 OUNCES

20 milliliters grapeseed oil

20 milliliters rose hip oil

10 milliliters apricot kernel oil

6 milliliters jojoba oil

10 drops grapefruit essential oil

2 droppers CBD oil (100 milligrams)

We used to be very skeptical of cleansing oil. Oil on already greasy skin? It sounded so counterintuitive that we avoided it altogether. On the other hand, the only other facial cleansers able to remove daily makeup and dirt left our skin dry and deprived. During one especially long winter, we opted for a cleansing oil and haven't looked back. Cleansing oils use the good oils to bind to and remove the bad oils, absorbing sebum and dirt directly from the skin. And since you rinse it off, along with the impurities of the day, it won't clog your pores—we promise.

1   Add all the ingredients in a 60-milliliter (2-ounce) pump bottle and gently shake to combine.

2   While your face is still dry, dispense a nickel-size amount of oil onto your fingertips and massage it into your skin. Rinse with warm water.

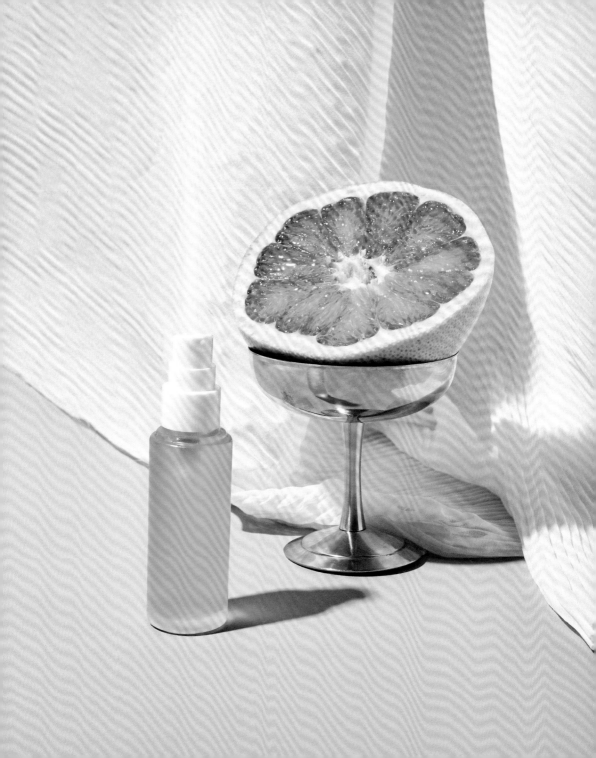

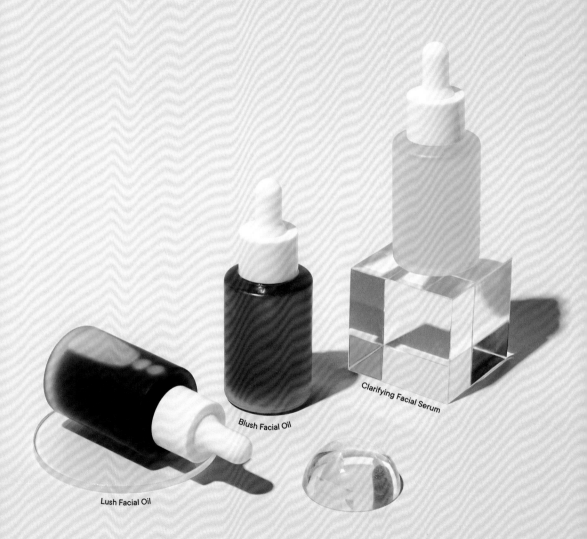

Lush Facial Oil

Blush Facial Oil

Clarifying Facial Serum

Clarifying Facial Serum

MAKES 1 OUNCE

10 milliliters vegetable glycerin

5 milliliters distilled water

1 tablespoon vitamin C powder

⅛ teaspoon hyaluronic acid powder

10 milliliters organic cold-pressed aloe vera gel

2 droppers CBD oil (100 milligrams)

½ tablespoon vitamin E oil

Serum is the middle child that doesn't get the attention it deserves. It should be applied in between cleansing and moisturizing since its smaller molecules will penetrate the skin deeper than your facial oil and help you maintain the moisture that is to come next. In this recipe, CBD and vitamin C team up to deliver a healthy dose of antioxidants to reduce inflammation and increase collagen production.

1   In a small bowl, combine the glycerin and water. Whisk in the vitamin C and hyaluronic acid powders until fully dissolved. One ingredient at a time, whisk in the aloe vera, CBD oil, and vitamin E until a smooth gel forms. Using a small funnel, pour the serum into a 30-milliliter (1-ounce) dropper bottle.

2   Shake before use and apply to the face and neck immediately after cleansing. Store in a cool, dark place to maintain the vitamin C's potency.

Fresh Face Facial Oils

MAKES 1 OUNCE

Everyone's skin has its dull days, caused by dehydration, lack of sleep, or changes in the weather. A few drops of facial oil will lock in moisture and restore your own natural oils. Our Blush recipe is ideal for dry or sensitive skin, packed full of gently nourishing ingredients like vitamin-rich carrot seed oil, with the floral scent of rose. For combination or oily skin, Lush is a lighter formula that regulates sebum production through quick-penetrating oils and fatty acids found in broccoli seed. Both recipes contain CBD, making either choice perfect for taming inflammation or treating skin conditions like eczema, rosacea, and acne. Apply after Clarifying Facial Serum (page 107).

Blush Facial Oil (for dry, sensitive skin)

5 milliliters grapeseed oil
5 milliliters pumpkin seed oil
5 milliliters chia seed oil
5 milliliters cranberry seed oil
5 milliliters rose hip oil

2 milliliters sea buckthorn oil
2 droppers CBD oil
   (100 milligrams)
1 milliliter carrot seed oil
5 drops rose essential oil

Lush Facial Oil (for combo or oily skin)

5 milliliters hemp seed oil
5 milliliters sunflower seed oil
5 milliliters marula oil
5 milliliters cucumber seed oil
5 milliliters apricot kernel oil
2 milliliters kukui nut oil

2 droppers CBD oil
   (100 milligrams)
1 milliliter broccoli seed oil
5 drops neroli essential oil
3 drops blue tansy essential oil

Combine all the ingredients for the desired variation in a 30-milliliter (1-ounce) dropper bottle. Shake well before using. Apply 5 to 10 drops to clean skin.

Face Masks

MAKES 1½ OUNCES

If you ask us, face masks are the most enjoyable part of self-care. The minor preparation process and gentle application is a relaxing ritual that lets you assess your skin's health and how best to treat it. Plus, a mask always leaves your skin soft and glowing. Our Strawberry Detoxifying Mask uses clay to draw out impurities and treat blackheads, whiteheads, and oversize pores. The Pumpkin Brightening Mask is a fall or winter favorite, introducing a pumpkin spice latte–inspired dose of vitamins and antioxidants to dry or dull skin. And our Honeydew-Lime Toning Mask is an all-star toner, tightening pores and providing the vitamin C essential for proper collagen production.

Strawberry Detoxifying Mask

1 tablespoon strawberry powder
1 tablespoon kaolin clay

1 tablespoon plain yogurt
¼ dropper CBD oil (12 milligrams)

Pumpkin Brightening Mask

2 tablespoons pumpkin puree
½ teaspoon oat milk
½ teaspoon honey (manuka, if you
    have it)

¼ dropper CBD oil (12 milligrams)
Pinch of ground cinnamon, ginger,
    allspice, and nutmeg (optional)

In a small bowl, combine all the ingredients for the desired variation. Apply the mask in an even layer to clean, dry skin and leave it on for 10 minutes. Rinse with warm water.

Honeydew-Lime Toning Mask

2 tablespoons crushed honeydew
   melon
1 teaspoon lime zest

1 teaspoon freshly squeezed lime
   juice
¼ dropper CBD oil (12 milligrams)

1   In a medium bowl, combine all the ingredients. With a fork, mash the mixture until smooth. Press the mixture through a fine mesh strainer (feel free to drink the drained juice!).

2   Apply the strained solids directly onto your face in a smooth layer. Leave it on for 10 minutes. Rinse with warm water. Avoid direct sunlight or use sunscreen within 24 hours of using the mask, as the brightening properties of citrus may cause sensitivity.

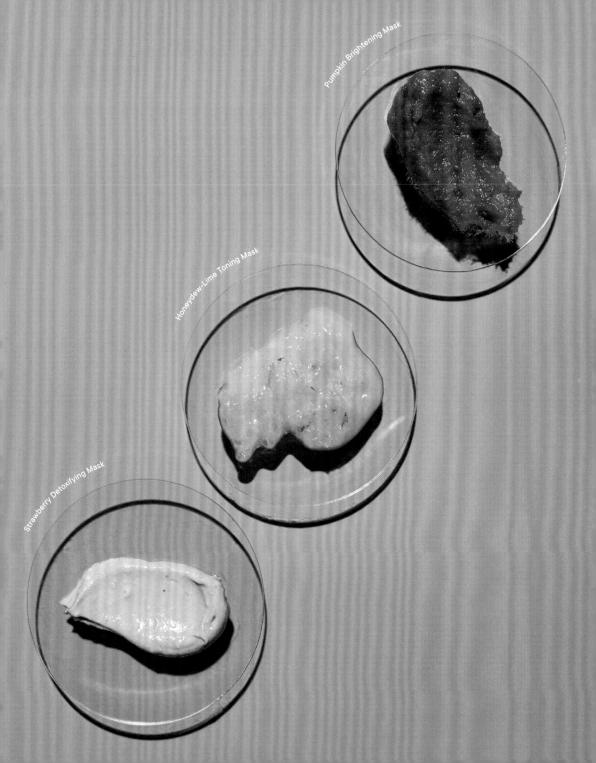

Pumpkin Brightening Mask

Honeydew-Lime Toning Mask

Strawberry Detoxifying Mask

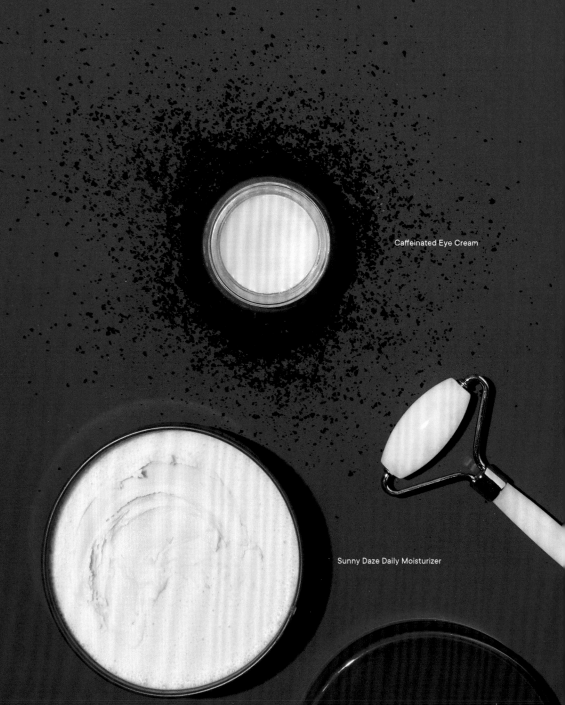

Caffeinated Eye Cream

Sunny Daze Daily Moisturizer

Sunny Daze Daily Moisturizer

MAKES 2 OUNCES

- 3 tablespoons shea butter
- 3 tablespoons sweet almond oil
- 1 teaspoon red raspberry seed oil
- 1 dropper CBD oil (50 milligrams)
- ¼ teaspoon non-nano zinc oxide powder
- 3 drops lemongrass essential oil

There is no greater defense against the signs of aging than the regular use of sunscreen. Protecting your face, neck, and chest from ultraviolet damage will help reduce dark spots, wrinkles, and other discoloration. While CBD itself will help regulate the renewal of skin cells when exposed to the sun, it's important that you apply SPF daily for protection from harsh rays. For further protection, we've added zinc oxide to our favorite moisturizer as well as red raspberry seed oil, which also contributes a surprisingly high level of SPF (between 28 and 50). A small dab on every exposed area of your skin will keep you looking young for years to come.

1   In a double boiler, or in a heatproof bowl set over a pan of simmering water, melt the shea butter, then add the almond and raspberry seed oils. Remove from the heat. Stir in the CBD oil, zinc oxide powder, and lemongrass oil, and mix until well combined. Refrigerate for 15 minutes or until the mixture is semisolid.

2   Using a hand mixer, whip the mixture until silky and creamy, 5 to 7 minutes. Scoop the moisturizer into a clean 2-ounce container with tight-fitting lid.

Caffeinated Eye Cream

MAKES 1 OUNCE

3 tablespoons rose
   hip oil
1 tablespoon fresh
   coffee beans or
   grounds
1 tablespoon beeswax
½ teaspoon jojoba oil
½ teaspoon vitamin
   E oil
3 drops geranium
   essential oil
1 dropper CBD oil
   (50 milligrams)

You're not alone if you wake up with dark circles or puffiness under your eyes. This is usually caused by a lack of sleep or dehydration, but allergies, PMS symptoms, or the tears from a bad breakup can have the same effect. This is the go-to cream to combat the swelling, infused with the energizing power of caffeine plus CBD to reduce inflammation. We chose geranium for its floral scent and added astringent properties, but lavender, rosemary, or bergamot are also fragrant and calming to the skin.

1   In a double boiler, or in a heatproof bowl set over a pan of simmering water, combine the rose hip oil and coffee beans and heat over low. Simmer for about 1 hour, stirring occasionally and adding more water to the base of the boiler as needed. Remove from the heat, let cool, then pour the mixture through cheesecloth or a paper towel into a small bowl or measuring cup.

2   Heat the double boiler again, this time melting the beeswax over low heat. Stir in the jojoba, vitamin E, geranium, and the coffee-infused oils.

3   Remove from the heat and stir in the CBD oil. Pour into a 30-milliliter (1-ounce) jar or container. Though not necessary, we like to store our cream in the refrigerator for an extra cooling effect when applied.

Manuka & Mint Lip Scrub

MAKES 1½ OUNCES

1 tablespoon cane
   sugar
1 tablespoon manuka
   honey
½ dropper CBD oil
   (25 milligrams)
2 drops peppermint
   essential oil

Keep your lips in mint condition by using this scrub two to three times per week. Besides CBD, the star ingredient here is manuka honey. Manuka contains antibacterial properties that regular honey lacks, and is recognized for its ability to treat just about anything—from healing cuts and scrapes to clearing infections and digestive issues when consumed. We chose manuka for this scrub because it is incredibly soothing when applied to the skin and is also unpasteurized (unlike grocery store honey) to maintain its natural properties. Raw honey, which is minimally processed as well, is a good substitute.

Cane sugar gives this scrub its texture, while CBD and peppermint oil join forces to provide an instant soothing and cooling sensation as you buff away dullness, uneven texture, and dry skin. You'll be left with soft lips that are prepped and ready for any lip color or occasion.

1 Mix all the ingredients in a small jar or a 60-milliliter (2-ounce) container.

2 Using a small spoon or cotton swab, scoop out a pea-size amount of scrub and apply directly to clean lips in circular motions to remove chapped skin. Wipe clean with a damp washcloth.

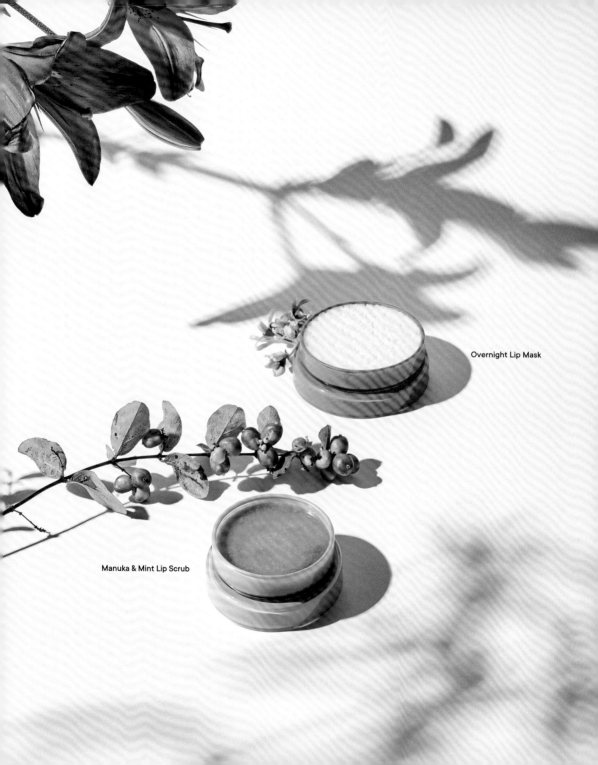

Overnight Lip Mask

Manuka & Mint Lip Scrub

Overnight Lip Mask

MAKES 2 OUNCES

2 tablespoons cupuaçu
butter

1 tablespoon coconut
oil

½ teaspoon candelilla
wax

¼ cup organic cold-
pressed aloe vera gel

2 droppers CBD oil
(100 milligrams)

5 drops lavender
essential oil

2 drops vanilla
essential oil

On days when the lip scrub and oil (pages 115 and 123) just don't seem to do the trick, an overnight mask can provide intense care for wind- or sun-damaged lips. With a higher concentration of CBD, this mask is designed to reduce the inflammation and associated pain. Aloe vera and cupuaçu butter (a vegan alternative to lanolin) also rejuvenate the affected skin and restore cell health by creating a blanket and barrier of moisture while you sleep. The sweet scent of lavender and vanilla offer up nighttime aromatherapy. Used weekly, this mask is an excellent component of a preventative skin care routine to ensure your lips are ready for anything.

1   In a small saucepan, melt the cupuaçu butter, coconut oil, and candelilla wax. Remove from the heat.

2   Slowly pour the aloe vera into the mixture while stirring continuously. Mix in the CBD and essential oils. Pour into a 60-milliliter (2-ounce) jar and let cool.

3   The mask should be thick and slightly gooey to the touch. Before bed, apply the mask with a cotton swab to coat the lips entirely.

Stress Spray

KEY BENEFITS:
Restores moisture, aromatherapy

MAKES 1 OUNCE

Spray stress away with a facial mist that doubles as a multipurpose hydrosol. Whether you're finishing a workout, prepping for a presentation, or waiting in line at the DMV, a refreshing spray is like a tall glass of cold water on a hot day. With CBD, each mist will tame redness, inflammation, and dryness while the essential oils provide further calm or energy.

Keep Calm

¼ cup rose hydrosol, homemade (recipe follows) or store-bought
1 tablespoon organic cold-pressed aloe vera gel

½ dropper CBD oil (25 milligrams)
2 teaspoons witch hazel
3 drops lavender essential oil

Keep Swimming

¼ cup cucumber hydrosol, homemade (recipe follows) or store-bought
1 tablespoon organic cold-pressed aloe vera gel

½ dropper CBD oil (25 milligrams)
2 teaspoons witch hazel
3 drops peppermint essential oil

1   To make the rose or cucumber hydrosol: Rinse 1 cup fresh rose petals or peel and slice 1 cup cucumber. In a large pot, combine the rose petals or cucumber slices along with just enough distilled water to cover. Bring to a boil, then simmer for 15 minutes. Strain through a sieve or cheesecloth and discard the solids. Let the hydrosol cool.

2   Combine all the ingredients for the desired variation in a 30-milliliter (1-ounce) bottle with a spray top or mister.

3   Spritz as often as needed on your face, body, or hair. We often make an extra batch without the CBD to use to freshen up the home, car, and even our gym bags.

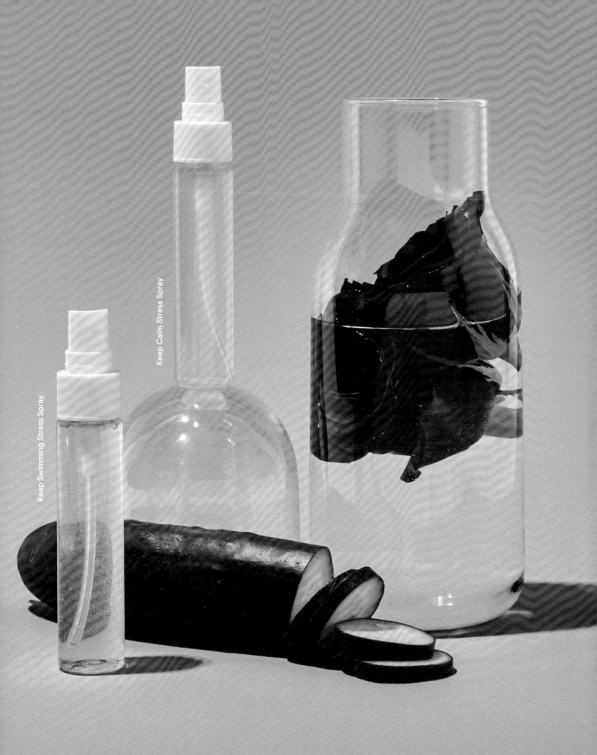

Keep Calm Stress Spray

Keep Swimming Stress Spray

Blemish Buster

MAKES 1 OUNCE

2 tablespoons organic cold-pressed aloe vera gel

12 drops tea tree oil

½ dropper CBD oil (25 milligrams)

TIPS:

- For a thicker mask, add 1 tablespoon of neem powder, which is recognized for its acne-healing properties and ability to reduce acne scars.
- Replace the aloe vera gel with ½ ounce (15 milliliters) witch hazel and mix together in a spray bottle for a full body application, or use as a facial toner. Shake well before each use.
- Apply our Sunny Daze Daily Moisturizer (page 113) after rinsing your face and before applying makeup. This lightweight emollient makes a perfect complement for oily and acne-prone skin.

There's nothing more relatable than the utter frustration of waking up with a pimple in the middle of your forehead. Stress, poor diet, or PMS often are the culprits of acne. Enter CBD to the rescue! As both an ingestible and topical remedy, CBD can combat pesky pimples with its anti-inflammatory properties and moderate the creation of sebum, the oily substance secreted by the skin. Paired with the antibacterial properties of tea tree oil and the anti-inflammatory effects of aloe vera, our blemish buster will work overnight to make sure your zits are zapped. P.S. This is also an effective treatment for bug bites!

In a 30-milliliter (1-ounce) jar or container, mix all the ingredients. Apply directly to blemishes with a clean cotton swab before bed. When you wake up, rinse your face with warm water.

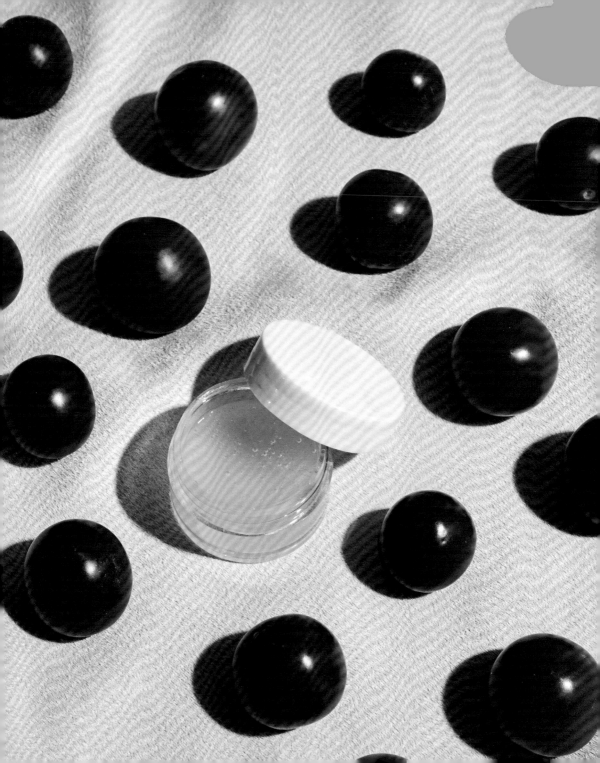

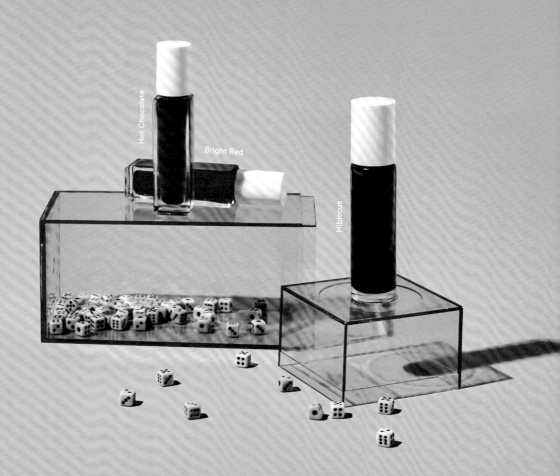

Hot Chocolate

Bright Red

Hibiscus

Hibiscus Lip Oil

MAKES 10 MILLILITERS

5 milliliters castor oil

2 milliliters sweet
almond oil

2 milliliters hibiscus
seed oil

1 dropper CBD oil
(50 milligrams)

2 drops ginger
essential oil

2 drops sweet orange
essential oil

¼ teaspoon hibiscus
flower powder

While glosses and balms create a barrier on the lips, lip oil's job is to absorb into the skin and provide hydration from within. We also love the way a lip oil adds color by blending flawlessly into your lip's natural texture without caking. In this recipe, we boost the soothing properties of CBD with hibiscus seed oil, a natural source of alpha hydroxy acids that support cell turnover. Along with a few drops of ginger, these oils also provide a slight plumping effect. For color, we doubled down on hibiscus for a universally flattering shade of rose, but there are plenty of botanical powders you can substitute and blend to create your perfect pigment.

Pour all the ingredients through a small funnel into a 10-milliliter roller bottle. Shake vigorously or use a toothpick to blend. Reapply frequently to maintain hydration and color.

OTHER NATURAL PIGMENTS:

- Bright Red: beetroot powder
- Moody Maroon: alkanet root powder
- Hot Chocolate: cocoa powder
- Peachy Nude: madder root powder
- Pretty in Pink: rose petal powder

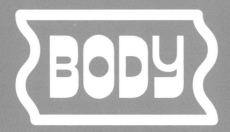

CBD has become a crucial part of total body health from the skin to within. While CBD oil can always be applied directly to areas experiencing pain, we've also found that pairing CBD with the right base and botanicals provides even greater coverage and effects. In smaller concentrations, CBD is excellent for all-over moisture and skin health as it takes on inflammation and dry-ness without mercy. CBD oil also fights free radicals to prevent signs of aging and can kill bacteria or deliver antioxidants to problem areas. With the right formulation and application, CBD can tackle a wide range of issues, from muscle pain to cellulite. These recipes are the source of some of our favorite whole body rituals. Self-Care Sunday, anyone?

Bath Soaks

There's no better ritual than a bath. For centuries, baths were considered a luxury, and it was only the rich or royal who could afford to bathe in privacy rather than at public bathhouses. Today, we continue to see baths as the epitome of self-care—a place where we can relax our minds and bodies in total comfort. It's no wonder you can find an endless supply of bath bombs and salts designed to detoxify, soothe, and restore. We've put together a few of our favorites, each containing a dose of CBD to target inflammation and irritation. Enjoy a soak post-workout or as part of your weekend ritual to keep your entire body in harmony.

MAKES 3 TO 6 BATH BOMBS, DEPENDING ON SIZE

Palo Santo Milk Bombs

1 cup baking soda
½ cup citric acid
½ cup coconut milk powder
1 dropper CBD oil (50 milligrams)

1 teaspoon fractionated coconut oil
10 drops palo santo essential oil
1 to 2 teaspoons water (if needed)

1   In a medium bowl, mix the baking soda, citric acid, and milk powder. Add the CBD, coconut, and palo santo oils. Mix well. Pinch a small handful—it should lightly clump. If not, add water ½ teaspoon at a time until the mixture holds together.

2   Shape the mixture into compact balls with your hands, or pack it into a bath bomb mold (a silicone ice cube tray also works). Let dry and store in an airtight container or shrink wrap for at least 24 hours.

3   Draw a warm bath, drop in a bomb, and sit back and relax.

Flower Power Tub Tea

1 cup rolled oats
½ cup sea salt
½ cup pink Himalayan salt
¼ cup dried lily flowers

¼ cup dried rosebuds
¼ cup dried jasmine flowers
¼ cup dried lavender
1 dropper CBD oil (50 milligrams)

1 In a medium bowl, mix all the ingredients. Distribute the mixture into muslin bags or fill a large tea infuser before each bath.

2 Draw a warm bath and drop a tea bag or infuser into the tub.

Total Detox Bath Salts

1 cup magnesium flakes
1 cup Dead Sea salt
½ cup pink Himalayan salt
½ cup bentonite clay
1 dropper CBD oil (50 milligrams)

1 teaspoon spirulina powder
10 drops lemon essential oil
5 drops eucalyptus essential oil
2 drops rosemary essential oil

1 In a medium bowl, mix all the ingredients. Transfer to and store in a large 24-ounce container with lid.

2 Pour 4 to 5 scoops or tablespoons of the salts into warm running water to dissolve.

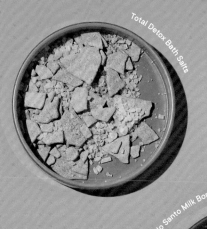

Total Detox Bath Salts

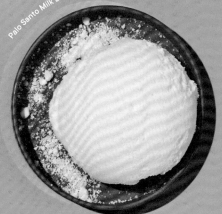

Palo Santo Milk Bomb

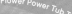

Flower Power Tub Tea

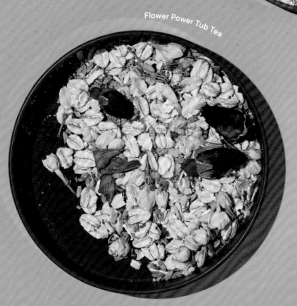

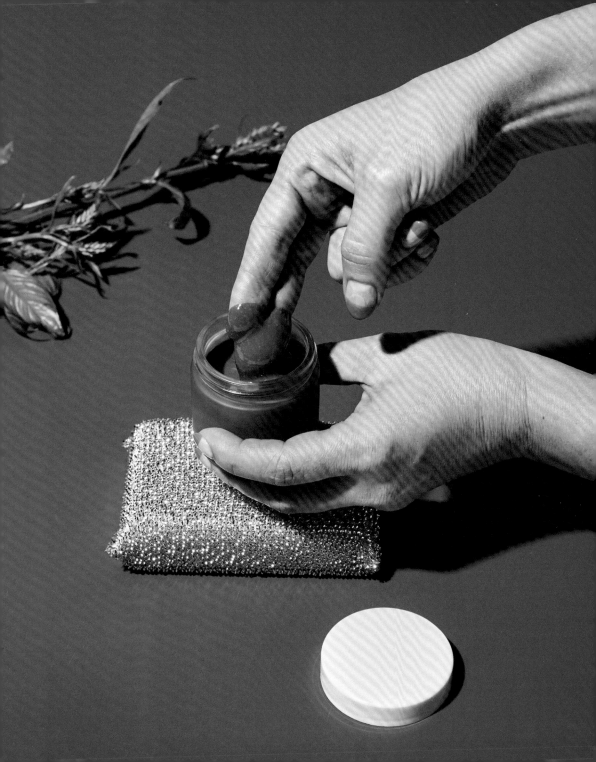

Leg & Booty Mask

KEY BENEFITS:
Plumps the skin
and clears pores

MAKES 2 OUNCES

¼ cup French green
  clay
2 tablespoons collagen
  powder
1 tablespoon green tea
  powder
1 dropper CBD oil
  (50 milligrams)
¼ cup vegetable
  glycerin

As we age, our skin loses elasticity, and our fat cells can become more prevalent along our thighs and booty. While exercise and a healthy diet will help combat the development of cellulite, this mask is a trusty sidekick whenever you notice an increase in bumps or lumps. Formulated with French green clay to draw out impurities, caffeine to dehydrate the fat cells, collagen to boost elasticity, and CBD to fight bacterial buildup, you'll be ready for any music video cameo that comes your way.

1   In a small bowl, combine the green clay and the collagen and green tea powders. Add the CBD oil and then slowly mix in the glycerin a few drops at a time. You want the mask to be thick and not drippy.

2   Lather over your backside and thighs. Pick two of your favorite booty jams and dance in your shower or bathtub for about 10 minutes or until the mask has hardened. Rinse or shower as usual.

Coconut Sugar Body Scrub

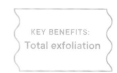

MAKES 8 OUNCES

1 cup coconut sugar
½ cup pink Himalayan salt
¼ cup fractionated coconut oil
2 droppers CBD oil (100 milligrams)

We'll be the first to admit that a sugar scrub was an overlooked product in our body routine for a long time. The first time we used one, we were sold. The right scrub not only exfoliates but also leaves you with a natural glow all over. Elbows, feet, even those little dips on either side of your ankles will be totally refreshed and silky smooth. In this recipe, we use both coconut sugar and pink Himalayan salt to remove dead skin from the surface, while CBD and coconut oils restore vital antioxidants to regenerate your cells. It takes just a few simple ingredients to promote circulation and moisture retention!

1   In a medium bowl, mix the sugar and salt, then add the coconut and CBD oils.

2   Using a hand mixer, whip the mixture to the desired consistency. Store in an 8-ounce jar with lid.

3   While you're showering, scoop a quarter-size amount into your hand and apply to rough areas in circular motions. Rinse and repeat until your entire body is smooth as silk.

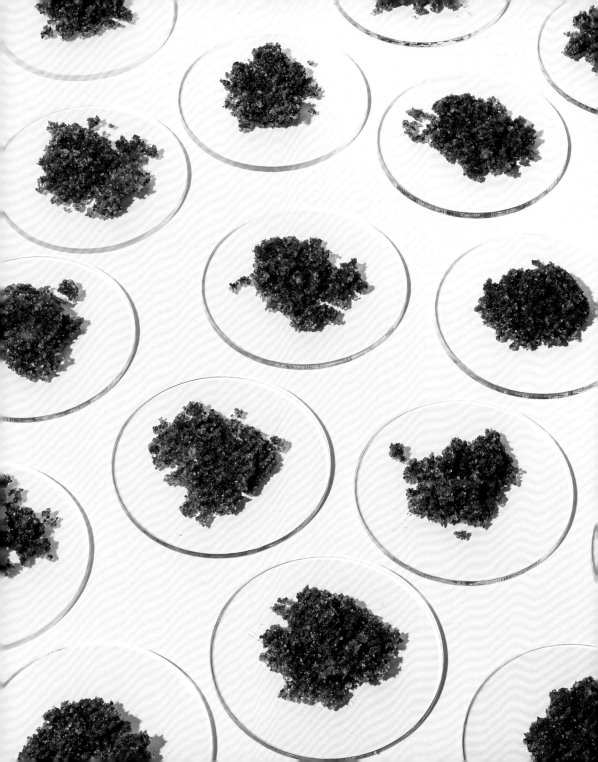

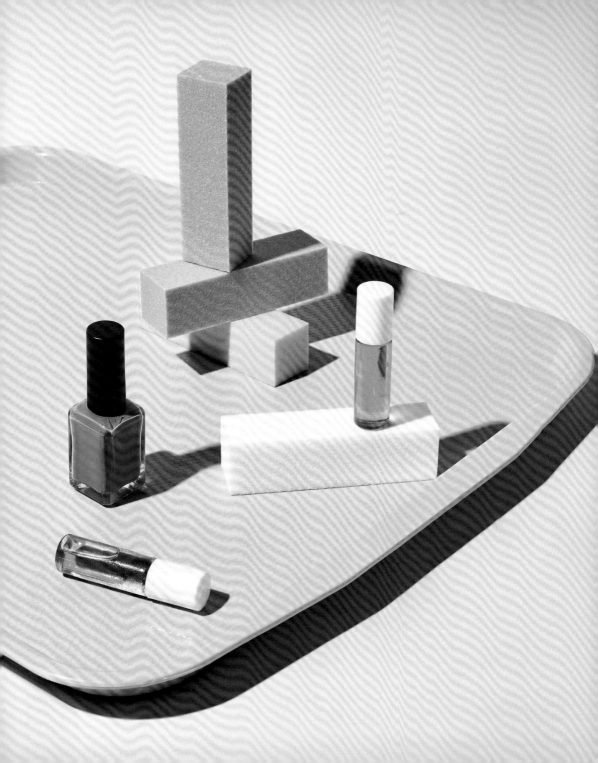

Cuticle Oil

MAKES 10 MILLILITERS

5 milliliters grapeseed
oil
4 milliliters avocado oil
½ dropper CBD oil
(25 milligrams)
10 drops carrot seed oil
10 drops vitamin E oil
5 drops frankincense
essential oil
3 drops lemon essential
oil
2 drops tea tree oil

The best way to give credit to your nail artist is to show off your stunning nails with cuticles to match. The combination of CBD with essential oils will strengthen your nail beds and heal cracked cuticles. Carrot seed and vitamin E, in particular, will fortify your nails, while tea tree and frankincense fight everyday bacteria. You never know when you might feel the urge to change careers and explore hand modeling.

1   Combine all the ingredients in a clean nail polish container, roller bottle, or cosmetic brush pen.

2   Apply along the cuticle line and across your nails (if they're not painted) twice per day. Don't forget your toenails!

Personal Lubricant

MAKES 1 OUNCE

15 milliliters cold-
pressed virgin
sunflower oil
10 milliliters, cold-
pressed virgin
apricot seed oil
5 milliliters calendula
oil
5 milliliters sweet
almond oil
1 dropper CBD oil
(50 milligrams)
2 drops peppermint
essential oil

IMPORTANT:

Oil-based lubes are not
latex-friendly. Oil can
degrade the integrity of
condoms, which could put
you and your partner at
risk for STIs or unintended
pregnancy. If you use latex
protection, look for a water-
or aloe-based lubricant
instead.

CBD is just as much for sexy time as it is for general wellness. Not only does the CBD oil decrease dryness and discomfort, but the sensual scent of calendula acts as an aphrodisiac. Some users find that CBD lube provides increased sensitivity, and most experience a feeling of relaxation that brings about a heightened sense of pleasure. Outside the bedroom, this lubricant can also be used to soothe postpartum pain or PMS symptoms—calendula's added antifungal and antibacterial properties boost the anti-inflammatory power of CBD. And yes, this oil is safe to ingest—that's why we add a few drops of peppermint.

Combine all the ingredients in a 30-milliliter (1-ounce) dropper or pump bottle. Apply a few drops as needed to soothe and lubricate.

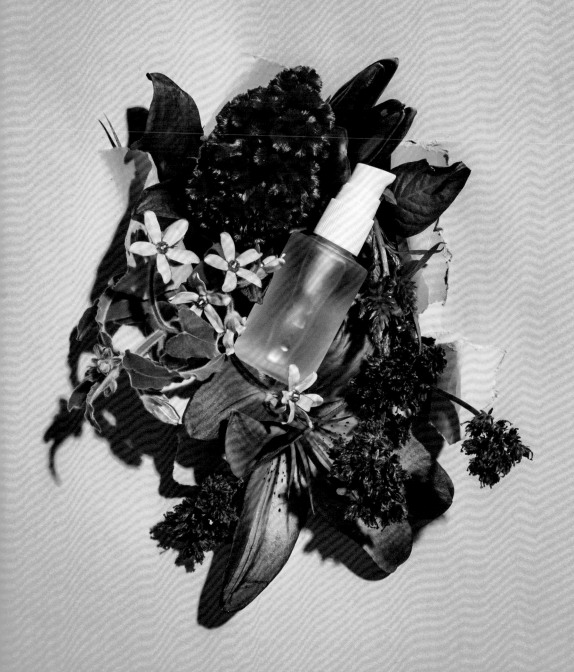

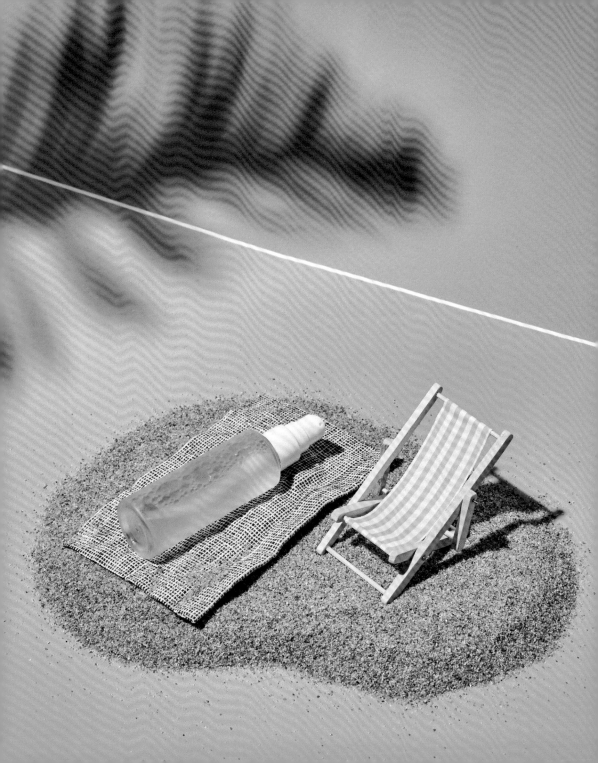

After-Sun Gel

KEY BENEFITS:
Relieves redness
and inflammation

MAKES 3 OUNCES

5 tablespoons organic
cold-pressed aloe
vera gel
4 droppers CBD oil
(200 milligrams)
10 drops vetiver
essential oil
10 drops sandalwood
essential oil
5 drops peppermint
essential oil
5 drops lavender
essential oil

NOTE:

Don't worry; the oil and aloe
separation is natural. Simply
shake before use.

As much as we try to religiously apply SPF, sometimes fun
in the sun results in a sunburn. Sunburns are the epitome of
inflammation, causing swelling and even blisters when rays are
too direct and strong. While there's no immediate cure for the
damage, aloe vera and CBD can play a major role in calming and
cooling the skin as it heals itself. Once your skin starts to peel
and shed the sun-damaged cells, this gel will continue to provide
antioxidants. We added essential oils of vetiver and sandalwood—
which may come as surprising choices. However, both essential
oils are centuries-old remedies to cool the body and calm the
mind. With its hit of peppermint, this after-sun gel will help lift
your spirits during a time of great physical discomfort and leave
you feeling refreshed every time.

1   Combine all the ingredients in a 90-milliliter (3-ounce) jar or pump
bottle.

2   Apply a thin layer directly on the affected area. Reapply only after
completely absorbed. For added relief during warm weather, soak
a washcloth in coconut water and a few drops of each essential oil.
Wring out and lay gently on top of the gel application to keep cool.

Crystal-Charged Body Oil

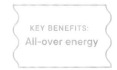
MAKES 2 OUNCES

Crystals of your choice
(see our favorites
below)
10 milliliters
fractionated coconut
oil
10 milliliters sunflower
seed oil
10 milliliters olive oil
10 milliliters jojoba oil
10 milliliters rose hip oil
6 milliliters argan oil
2 droppers CBD oil
(100 milligrams)
10 drops cedarwood
essential oil
10 drops frankincense
essential oil
4 drops ylang-ylang
essential oil
4 drops mandarin
essential oil

Ancient Egyptians are said to be among the first people to have used crystals to ward off illness and negative energy. Since then, healing with crystals has evolved throughout many cultures. Each type of crystal is associated with its own power and allows for positive energy to flow into the body, making them a perfect addition for an all-over CBD body oil.

1   Before making this recipe, dedicate some time for inward reflection and, based on your current emotional or physical state, choose the crystal that calls to you. Once you've selected your crystal, purchase one small enough to fit in your chosen container. Alternatively, if you can't find small crystals, infuse the oil in a large widemouthed jar and transfer it to a pump dispenser bottle.

2   Put the crystals in the container, pour all the ingredients over them, and mix or shake to combine.

3   You can use this oil at any time, but you'll get maximum absorption when your skin is clean and fresh. We recommend applying the oil liberally right after a bath or shower.

A FEW OF OUR FAVORITE CRYSTALS:

- Clear quartz: Sets intention and brings positive energy
- Rose quartz: Brings love and emotional healing
- Black tourmaline: Removes negative energy
- Amethyst: Provides protection and peace
- Citrine: Promotes manifestation and motivation
- Jasper: Aligns chakras and balances yin/yang energies
- Fluorite: Inspires clarity and relaxation
- Green jade: Brings abundance and prosperity

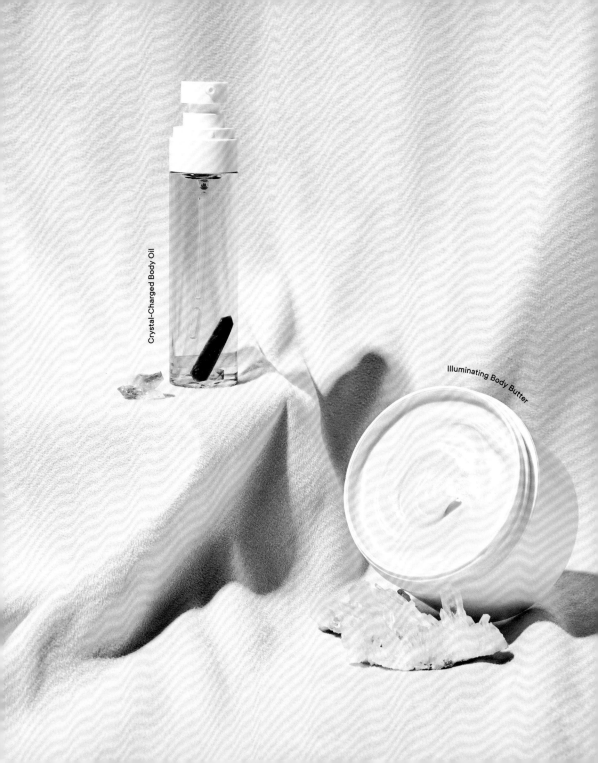

Crystal-Charged Body Oil

Illuminating Body Butter

Illuminating Body Butter

MAKES 8 OUNCES

¼ cup organic refined
coconut oil

¼ cup organic refined
shea butter

¼ cup cocoa butter

¼ cup sunflower oil

2 droppers CBD oil
(100 milligrams)

5 drops jasmine
essential oil

5 drops grapefruit
essential oil

¼ teaspoon lab-created
mica powder (we
like gold and pearl
pigments)

This is a go-to recipe when you're ready to light up a room. Coconut oil, shea butter, and cocoa butter act as a triple threat, rich in fatty acids to nourish your skin and improve elasticity while creating a moisture barrier that ensures skin free from dry spots. These luxurious butters are then whipped with CBD and mica to create a shimmery cream that leaves your skin soft and glowing.

1 In a double boiler, or in a heatproof bowl set over a pan of simmering water, melt the coconut oil, shea butter, and cocoa butter. Remove from the heat, pour into a medium bowl, and let cool for 5 minutes.

2 Stir in the sunflower, CBD, and essential oils and the mica powder, and continue to let cool (or refrigerate) until the edges start to harden—about 1 hour.

3 Once the mixture looks a little cloudy, whip it with a hand mixer until thick and fluffy, about 8 minutes. Refrigerate for 3 to 5 minutes to let it set and then transfer to jars or other containers.

Cramp Cream

MAKES 6 OUNCES

½ cup magnesium
  flakes
1 tablespoon boiling
  water
¼ cup coconut oil
3 tablespoons shea
  butter
2 tablespoons
  emulsifying wax
4 droppers CBD oil
  (200 milligrams)
10 drops peppermint
  essential oil
10 drops clary sage
  essential oil
5 drops thyme
  essential oil
5 drops ylang-ylang
  essential oil

Monthly hormone imbalance, skin breakouts, and unhealthy food cravings are bad enough, but cramps really are the last straw. PMS cramps can be debilitating and painful; luckily, our Cramp Cream is here to provide relief. Its key ingredients, magnesium and CBD, help decrease pain and stiffness from within, while clary sage and peppermint calm bloating. So settle into a binge-a-thon, sip some chamomile tea, and rub this cream onto your lower abdomen and back as often as needed.

1   Put the magnesium flakes in a small bowl and add the boiling water to dissolve them. You should have a thick liquid. Set aside to cool.

2   In a double boiler, or in a heatproof bowl set over a pan of simmering water, melt the coconut oil, shea butter, and emulsifying wax. Pour the mixture into a bowl and let cool to room temperature.

3   Using a hand mixer, blend the CBD and essential oils into the coconut oil mixture. Slowly add the magnesium liquid a few drops at a time. Continue mixing until well blended.

4   Refrigerate for 15 minutes to chill. Blend the mixture once more to a buttery consistency and scoop into a 180-milliliter (6-ounce) container. Store in the refrigerator for an added cooling sensation when applied.

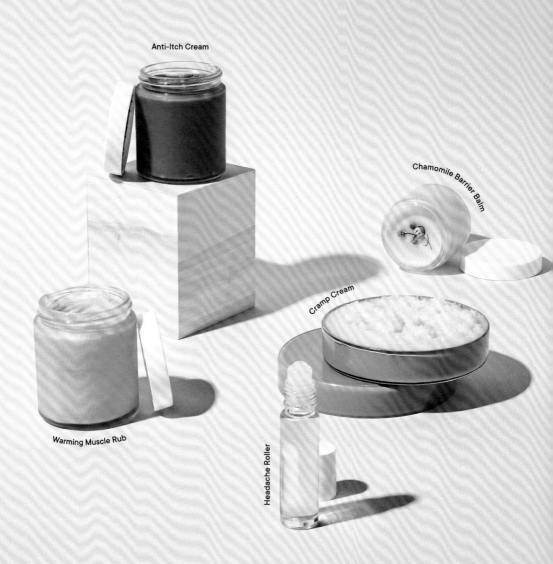

Anti-Itch Cream

Chamomile Barrier Balm

Cramp Cream

Warming Muscle Rub

Headache Roller

Warming Muscle Rub

MAKES 4 OUNCES

⅓ cup raw cocoa butter
⅓ cup beeswax
¼ cup coconut oil
1 teaspoon cayenne
  pepper
4 droppers CBD oil
  (200 milligrams)
10 drops peppermint
  essential oil
5 drops camphor
  essential oil
5 drops ginger
  essential oil

While we always recommend a good stretch to help relieve the pain and stiffness of sore muscles, sometimes it's not enough. To increase blood circulation and release tension, this warming muscle rub is infused with cayenne, CBD, and ginger. Capsaicin, the active ingredient in cayenne, helps block pain transmitters, while CBD and ginger work together to ease inflammation and swelling. A few drops of peppermint and camphor essential oils help boost circulation and provide an initial cooling sensation that gives way to a warmer feeling. For added relief, our Total Detox Bath Salts (page 126) are a great way to relax your muscles.

1   In a double boiler, or in a heatproof bowl set over a pan of simmering water, melt the cocoa butter, beeswax, and coconut oil. Add the cayenne and mix until completely dissolved.

2   Remove from the heat and mix in the CBD and essential oils. Pour into a 120-milliliter (4-ounce) jar or multiple smaller containers and let cool.

3   Apply a small amount to the affected area and rub it in gently. Your skin may become slightly red—from the ingredients' coloring—and you'll feel a pleasant warming sensation. Wash your hands afterward and avoid contact with your eyes and other sensitive body parts.

Headache Roller

MAKES 10 MILLILITERS

8 milliliters jojoba oil
2 droppers CBD oil
(100 milligrams)
10 drops lavender
essential oil
10 drops peppermint
essential oil
5 drops frankincense
essential oil

TIP:

You can find roller bottles online and in many stores that carry essential oils. We prefer the kind with glass or stainless-steel (rather than plastic) balls because they seem to get stuck less and also offer a light cooling sensation when applied.

Headaches are the results of intense stimulation to sensory nerves—a response to inflammatory agents released when pain or a migraine occurs. They can knock you down fast, but over-the-counter painkillers have their undesirable side effects too. While ingesting CBD helps regulate and decrease inflammation throughout the body as a preventative treatment, this one-hundred-milligram CBD roller is handy for unexpected pain. You won't waste any time kicking a headache to the curb! The high concentration of CBD will target tension and inflammation, while the menthol in the peppermint oil will help your muscles relax even further. The lavender and frankincense complete the blend, soothing your senses and allowing your mind to slip into a state of relaxation.

1   Combine all the ingredients in a 10-milliliter glass roller bottle with a stainless-steel ball. Shake gently to combine.

2   At the onset of a headache, roll directly on your temples and at the base of your neck and shoulders, where tension is greatest. We also like to do a small roll underneath the nose to let aromatherapy take over. If you can, close your eyes and lie down somewhere dark until the headache subsides. You can even use this blend (without the jojoba and CBD) in an essential oil diffuser to enhance the aromatherapy effects.

Chamomile Barrier Balm

MAKES 2 OUNCES

2 tablespoons organic beeswax pellets

2 tablespoons coconut oil

1 tablespoon olive oil

1 dropper CBD oil (50 milligrams)

10 drops chamomile essential oil

5 drops lavender essential oil

5 drops clary sage essential oil

2 drops bergamot essential oil

TIP:

You can easily transform this recipe into a slightly less firm lip balm by replacing the olive oil with shea butter and doubling the amount of coconut oil. To add color, add ½ teaspoon of your favorite floral powder—like hibiscus, rose, alkanet—or lab-created mica.

Protect yourself against the elements with our barrier balm, perfect for dry patches or areas of intense inflammation. With just enough give to glide across the skin, this balm will stay in place without feeling greasy. This is our favorite for tired or tense muscles in the neck or lower back and serves as a great protector against wind and dry air when applied to your lips.

1   In a double boiler, or in a heatproof bowl set over a pan of simmering water, melt the beeswax and coconut oil until liquefied. Stir in the olive oil and remove from the heat. Add the CBD and essential oils and mix well.

2   Pour the mixture into a widemouthed container or paper push tube (similar to a lip balm tube) and let cool completely. Apply a small amount or rub the tube across areas that need extra protection, such as elbows, feet, or lower back.

Anti-Itch Cream

MAKES 4 OUNCES

⅓ cup bentonite clay
¼ cup witch hazel
¼ cup vegetable
   glycerin
3 tablespoons raw
   honey
2 droppers CBD oil
   (100 milligrams)
2 milliliters calendula
   oil
10 drops tea tree oil
5 drops frankincense
   essential oil
5 drops lavender
   essential oil

It takes an extreme amount of willpower to resist an itch. Whether caused by mosquitos, allergies, or eczema, rashes and irritation are almost impossible to ignore. This thick cream steps in to mediate, delivering antiseptic and cleansing properties via powerful ingredients like witch hazel, clay, and raw honey. CBD steps in to help reduce inflammation and swelling, and the essential oils of tea tree, frankincense, and lavender each play their role to calm and soothe the skin. Apply whenever you feel the urge to scratch.

1   In a small bowl, combine the bentonite clay, witch hazel, vegetable glycerin, honey, CBD oil, and calendula oil. Mix until smooth and then add the essential oils. Mix again to create a paste-like consistency. If it's too thick, add more vegetable glycerin or distilled water, a few drops at a time. Pour the mixture into a 120-milliliter (4-ounce) container with lid.

2   For rashes or bug bites, apply the lotion to cover the affected areas as needed.

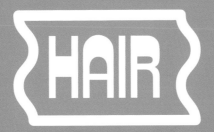

Is it really that surprising that the research involving CBD's effects on hair is yielding positive results? In the same way that CBD nourishes and protects our skin, it can perform the same wonders for our hair and scalp. CBD contains antioxidants and amino acids, the building blocks for protein, giving it the ability to prevent breakage and strengthen hair while also protecting it against free radicals and environmental stressors like pollution and smoke. It also contains fatty acids to help promote hair growth and regulates sebum (or oil), making it ideal for all hair types. Even CBD's anti-inflammatory nature can save a dry, itchy scalp so you don't have to hide those locks under a beanie all winter long. Bottom line: if you're dreaming of thick hair and a healthy scalp, these recipes are your new BFF.

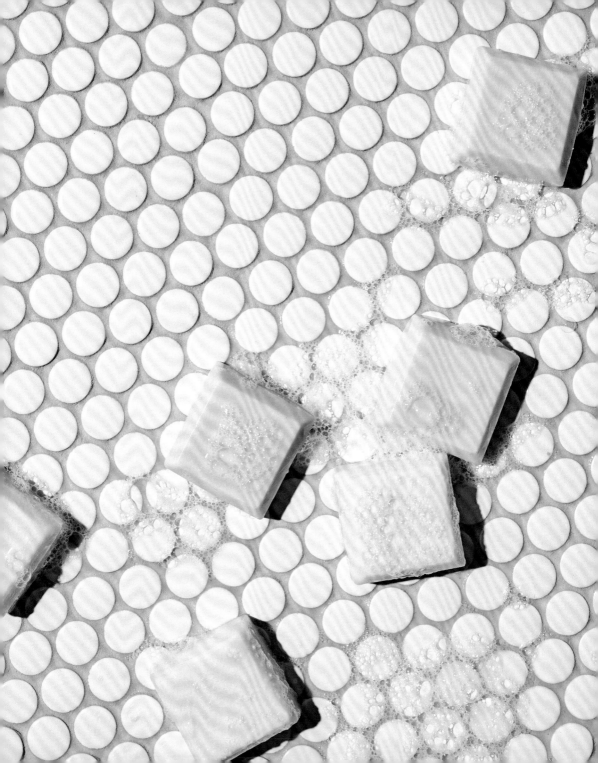

Coconut Colada Shampoo & Conditioner Bars

MAKES 4 TO 6 BARS, DEPENDING ON SIZE

Shampoo and conditioner labels have always been difficult to decipher aside from the primary ingredient always listed first: water. These bars are different. Blended with botanicals and concentrated without water, they're a travel-friendly alternative that will keep your hair clean and hydrated. If Coconut Colada isn't your favorite scent, we've included alternative essential oil blends by hair type. Simply replace the lime with the essential oil of your choice.

Shampoo

¼ cup mango butter
¼ cup melt-and-pour glycerin base or liquid castile soap

½ cup coconut milk
1 dropper CBD oil (50 milligrams)
5 drops lime essential oil

Conditioner

½ cup cocoa butter
⅓ cup mango butter
⅓ cup shea butter

2 tablespoons beeswax
1 dropper CBD oil (50 milligrams)
5 drops lime essential oil

1   In a double boiler, or in a heatproof bowl set over a pan of simmering water, melt the mango butter and glycerin base (shampoo) or all the butters and beeswax (conditioner) together. Remove from the heat and gently stir in the remaining ingredients.

2   Pour into a mold of your choice. Wood boxes, silicone molds, cupcake tins, and even ice cube trays are great for creating these vacation-ready bars.

3   To use, rub the bar between your palms to work up a slight lather, then apply to your scalp and strands. Be sure to massage! Rinse with warm water.

ESSENTIAL OILS BY HAIR TYPE:

- Oily hair: bergamot, eucalyptus, peppermint, clary sage, cedarwood
- Thinning hair: rosemary, rosewood, lemongrass, cedarwood, grapefruit
- Dry scalp: geranium, rosemary, tea tree, patchouli, lavender
- Dry, dull hair: ylang-ylang, geranium, rose
- Frizzy hair: ylang-ylang, lavender

Dry Scalp Elixir

KEY BENEFITS:
Heals and prevents
dryness and irritation

MAKES 1 OUNCE

10 milliliters avocado oil
5 milliliters coconut oil
5 milliliters olive oil
5 milliliters argan oil
3 milliliters hemp
  seed oil
2 droppers CBD oil
  (100 milligrams)
10 drops tea tree oil
5 drops lemon
  essential oil
5 drops rosemary
  essential oil

As if dry skin wasn't enough, it's even worse when the itching and flaking comingle on top of your head. A weekly treatment during flare-ups or winter months will keep your scalp nourished and moisturized. This elixir contains fatty oils and the antioxidant power of CBD, along with clarifying essential oils to fight bacteria and residue. We tend to use this elixir once a week during the dry months of winter and less frequently during other seasons, though it's also an excellent treatment for recovering from sunburns if you forget to add SPF to your hair part.

1   Combine all the ingredients in a 30-milliliter (1-ounce) dropper bottle. Shake gently to combine.

2   Part your hair in sections and use the dropper to apply the elixir until you have covered your entire scalp. Massage the elixir in thoroughly with your fingertips and leave on for 10 minutes. For exceptional dryness, apply the elixir, wrap your head in plastic wrap, and leave on for 20 minutes.

3   Rinse and style as usual.

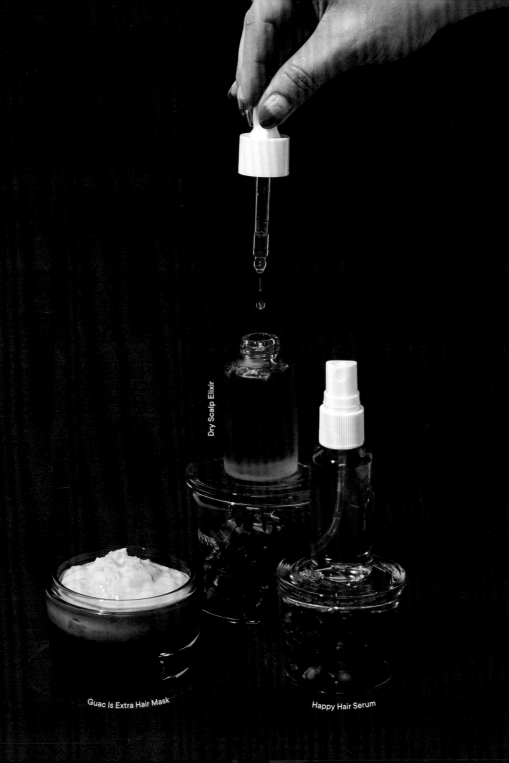

Dry Scalp Elixir

Guac Is Extra Hair Mask

Happy Hair Serum

Guac Is Extra Hair Mask

MAKES 6 OUNCES

½ ripe avocado
½ cup coconut milk
2 tablespoons honey
2 droppers CBD oil
(100 milligrams)

Guacamole on the side may cost extra, but it's always worth it. The same goes for this ultraconditioning hair mask, where avocado is the star ingredient, nourishing your scalp and hair follicles as it repairs and prevents damage. Rich in fatty amino acids, vitamins (A, B6, D, and E), and minerals (iron and copper), the mask also features coconut milk, honey, and CBD in supporting roles to provide moisture that fights frizz and strengthens your locks.

1 Combine all the ingredients in a medium bowl and blend with a hand mixer or immersion blender until smooth.

2 Separate your hair into sections and apply the mask, massaging it into your hair and scalp with a circular motion. Cover with a shower cap or plastic wrap and use a hairdryer to heat your hair for about 15 minutes. Or, if the sun is shining, grab a book and sit under the warm rays for 30 minutes. If you don't have a hairdryer or a sunny sky, leave the mask on for 1 hour.

3 Rinse and wash your hair as usual. Repeat weekly or as needed.

Happy Hair Serum

MAKES ½ OUNCE

5 milliliters argan oil
5 milliliters sweet
  almond oil
4 milliliters rose hip oil
1 dropper CBD oil
  (50 milligrams)
2 drops honeysuckle
  essential oil
2 drops bergamot
  essential oil
1 drop grapefruit
  essential oil
1 drop gardenia
  essential oil

If you want your hair to shine, you've come to the right recipe. Along with CBD, we tested for other oils that give the most luster without the weight so that this finishing serum could protect against UV and heat damage while staying soft to the touch. The combined forces of argan, sweet almond, and rose hip oils will make it look like you've been photoshopped for a hair commercial, while the bright scents of honeysuckle, bergamot, grapefruit, and gardenia invigorate your mood.

1 Combine all the ingredients in a 15-milliliter (½-ounce) pump or spray bottle.

2 Shake well before use. Apply a few drops to wet hair before using styling tools or smooth on dry hair to touch up flyaways.

Baby Got Beard Oil

MAKES 1 OUNCE

10 milliliters jojoba oil

10 milliliters coconut oil

5 milliliters argan oil

3 milliliters cranberry seed oil

2 droppers CBD oil (100 milligrams)

5 drops sandalwood essential oil

5 drops neroli essential oil

2 drops clary sage essential oil

Most beard oils fail to find a scent that's universally appealing. Blends either lean toward smoky or fruity without many neutral options. This beard oil bats right down the center with a light woodsy scent complemented by mellow citrus. Of course, you can always add other essential oils to your liking, but don't skip the cranberry seed and CBD oils. Cranberry contains omega-3 fatty acids and vitamin E, which make it a great conditioner that absorbs without feeling greasy.

1   Combine all the ingredients in a 30-milliliter (1-ounce) dropper bottle.

2   After cleansing, use only a few drops for a mustache and up to ¼ dropper for beards—a little goes a long way. Dispense directly onto the hair and comb through. Style as usual.

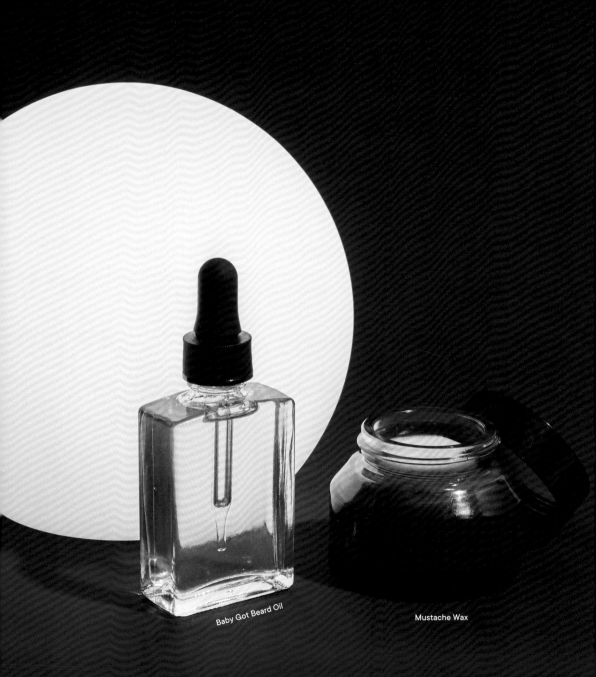

Baby Got Beard Oil

Mustache Wax

Mustache Wax

MAKES 2 OUNCES

¼ cup beeswax
  pastilles
2 tablespoons shea
  butter
1 dropper CBD oil
  (50 milligrams)
2 tablespoons argan oil
15 drops cedarwood
  essential oil
5 drops ginger
  essential oil

Not only does wax define and hold the shape of your mustache, but CBD-infused wax coats your follicles to offer protection and nourishment. Both argan oil and CBD are high in antioxidant content and fatty acids to restore moisture and protect against the elements, ensuring a 'stache that's soft and smooth. For the scent, we chose a slightly spicy, woodsy blend of cedarwood and ginger but always recommend using essential oils you want to smell on the daily.

1   In a double boiler, or in a heatproof bowl set over a pan of simmering water, melt the beeswax and shea butter.

2   Remove from the heat and add the CBD, argan, and essential oils. Pour into a 60-milliliter (2-ounce) container or jar with lid and let cool.

3   To style, rub a small amount between your fingers to heat up. Apply to mustache or beard.

Texturizing Salt Spray

MAKES 4 OUNCES

1 cup coconut water
1 tablespoon sea salt
½ tablespoon coconut
  sugar
½ dropper CBD oil
  (25 milligrams)
5 drops bergamot
  essential oil
5 drops sandalwood
  essential oil

With CBD's power to strengthen hair, an everyday salt spray is an easy way to add definition and protection. Paired with coconut water and coconut sugar, and full of essential vitamins and minerals like vitamin C and potassium, this fragrant spray will also condition each strand to prevent breakage. Smoother locks, less frizz, and moisture-rich follicles—you'll feel and smell like you're on a tropical vacation.

1 In a small saucepan, heat the coconut water over low heat. Add the salt and sugar and stir until dissolved.

2 Remove from the heat and add the oils, mixing to combine. Pour the mixture into a 120-milliliter (4-ounce) spray bottle and let cool.

3 Shake well before using. Spritz onto your hair while it is still damp. Scrunch or twirl hair with your fingers to define and shape. You may also lightly spray after curling your hair, but be careful not to oversaturate and dampen your curls.

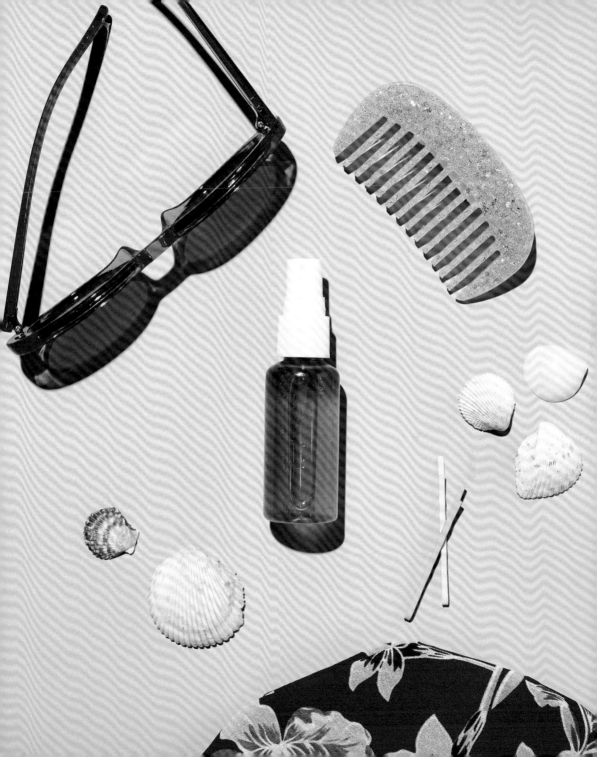

High Brow Primer

MAKES 10 MILLILITERS

5 milliliters organic
cold-pressed aloe
vera gel
4 milliliters castor oil
½ dropper CBD oil
(25 milligrams)

TIPS:

· Add a tint of color to
your brows by adding a
matching pigment. Slowly
add ⅛ teaspoon cocoa
or charcoal powder (to
prevent clumping) until
you reach your desired
color.

· Switch the ratio of aloe
vera to castor oil to adjust
the consistency for your
eyelashes—remember to
do a patch test to avoid
irritated eyes!

This primer will take you from low brow to high brow in less than thirty seconds. While aloe vera grooms your brows to keep them in line, the castor and CBD oils coat the follicles to thicken and promote growth. They'll become softer to the touch and hold their shape while you hold your own.

In a small bowl or jar, combine all the ingredients and mix well. Using a small funnel, pour the primer into a 10-milliliter mascara tube. Use the wand to apply to your brows and hold the perfect shape.

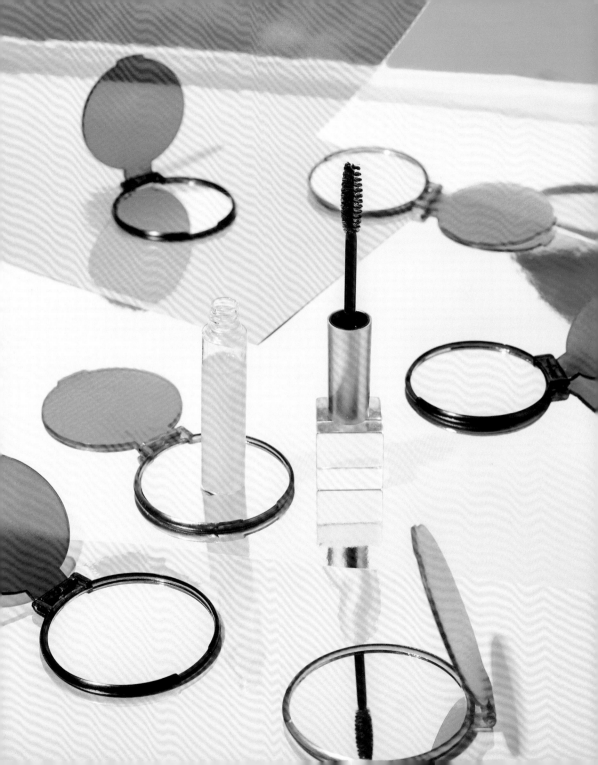

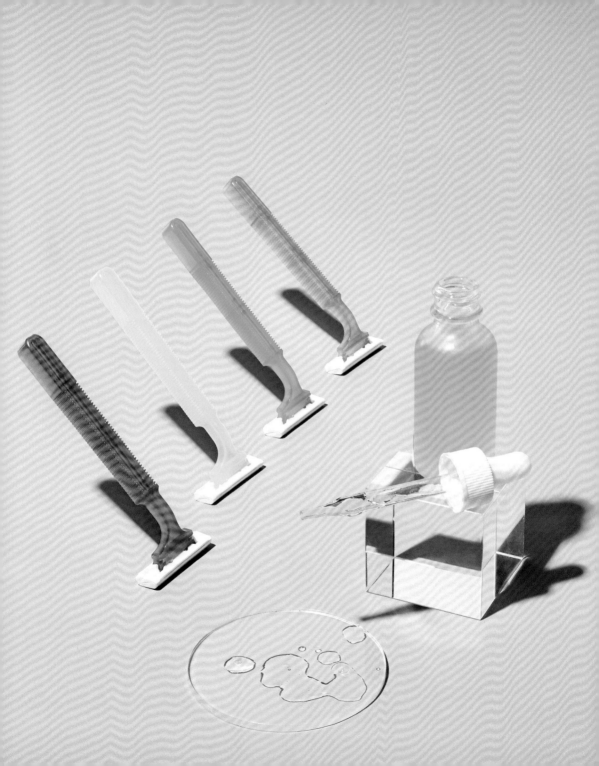

Ingrown Eliminator

KEY BENEFITS:
Prevents redness and
reduces inflammation

MAKES 1 OUNCE

15 milliliters jojoba oil

13 milliliters grapeseed
oil

2 droppers CBD oil
(100 milligrams)

10 drops peppermint
essential oil

5 drops clove essential
oil

5 drops tea tree oil

5 drops eucalyptus
essential oil

5 drops lavender
essential oil

5 drops clary sage
essential oil

5 drops lemon essential
oil

Say goodbye to razor burn and bikini line bumps with this oil made for ingrown hair. A blend of antimicrobial essential oils and moisturizing seed oils soothe irritation and redness while ensuring that each pore is clear and clean. CBD, in particular, helps tackle inflammation, keeping those pesky red bumps from ever rising above the surface. We highly recommend keeping a travel size handy for vacations and long summer weekends.

1   Combine all the ingredients in a 30-milliliter (1-ounce) dropper bottle and shake to combine.

2   After shaving or waxing, apply a few drops directly to wherever you shaved and gently massage into the skin until absorbed. Follow with your favorite body oils or lotions.

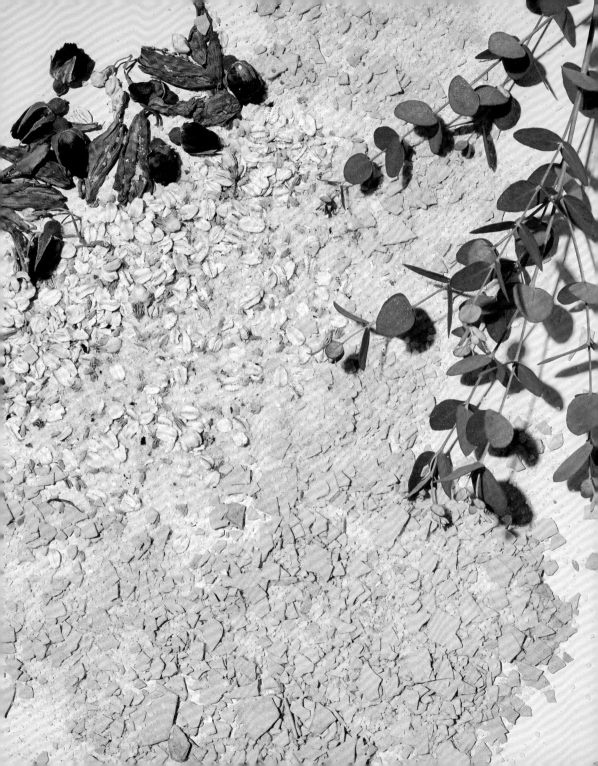

ACKNOWLEDGMENTS

Chris and I met while studying Shakespeare during a summer abroad in London, and while we've always been avid writers, it's safe to say we never expected CBD to be the topic of our first published work. We have so many people to thank for supporting us not only with this book but in every way imaginable since Dazey was founded.

First, we have to thank our cofounders and best friends, Scott and Emily. Thank you for helping us build a brand and style that is uniquely Dazey. We're eternally grateful to the higher powers that our camping spot happened to be next to yours at the Sasquatch Music Festival in 2016. Thank you to our respective families, who have encouraged us and shared Dazey with their friends. Thank you to each of our friends who do the same.

Of course, we have to say thank you to our editors, Jennifer Worick and Bridget Sweet, for believing we should even author a book and for guiding us through the entire process until every page was just right. To our creative team—Tony Ong, Lauren Segal, and Mandy Kehoe—we are so appreciative of your eyes for design that brought our brand to life in print, and to Kayla Wakayama of Juniper Nail Bar for making sure our nails looked as fly as the recipes.

Last, but certainly not least, thank you to our customers and to all you CBD fans. The future of hemp is extremely bright, and we have so much to look forward to together. Your stories and feedback inspire our work (and recipes!) every day. We hope you continue to share your experiences with others and destigmatize CBD in the workplace and everyday life.

—Tori Bodin

NOTES

1   http://druglibrary.org/schaffer/hemp/history/first12000/3.htm

2   www.leafly.com/news/cannabis–101/where-did-the-word-marijuana-come
-from-anyway–01fb

3   Ibid.

4   www.druglibrary.org/schaffer/hemp/taxact/mjtaxact.htm

5   https://ministryofhemp.com/hemp/history

6   Ibid.

7   Ibid.

8   www.congress.gov/bill/113th-congress/house-bill/2642

9   www.agriculture.senate.gov/2018–farm-bill

10   www.leafly.com/news/cannabis–101/what-is-cbg-cannabinoid

11   www.ncbi.nlm.nih.gov/pubmed/19112869

12   www.ncbi.nlm.nih.gov/pubmed/23415610

13   www.ncbi.nlm.nih.gov/pubmed/25252936

14   www.ncbi.nlm.nih.gov/pubmed/25269802

15   www.ncbi.nlm.nih.gov/pubmed/18681481

16   www.ncbi.nlm.nih.gov/pubmed/23415610

17   www.ncbi.nlm.nih.gov/pubmed/26197538

18   www.leafly.com/news/cannabis–101/what-is-cannabichromene-cbc
-cannabinoid

19   www.leafly.com/news/science-tech/what-is-cbn-and-what-are-the
-benefits-of-this-cannabinoid

20   www.ncbi.nlm.nih.gov/pubmed/22038065

21   https://lpi.oregonstate.edu/mic/dietary-factors/phytochemicals/chlorophyll
-chlorophyllin#disease-prevention

22   www.mayoclinic.org/drugs-supplements-vitamin-e/art–20364144

23   www.leafly.com/news/cannabis–101/terpenes-the-flavors-of-cannabis
-aromatherapy

24   Ibid.

25   www.fda.gov/news-events/press-announcements/statement-consumer
-warning-stop-using-thc-vaping-products-amid-ongoing-investigation-lung
-illnesses

GLOSSARY

Key Superfoods and Beauty Ingredients

ALOE VERA GEL: An emollient obtained from aloe vera leaves that has hydrating, healing, antimicrobial, and anti-inflammatory properties. It has a slightly relaxing effect on the skin, making it ideal for sensitive, sunburned, and sun-exposed skin.

APRICOT KERNEL OIL: A nongreasy emollient rapidly absorbed by the skin and high in vitamin E. Often used as a substitute for almond oil.

ARGAN OIL: From the nut of the argan tree, this oil protects and moisturizes the skin.

ASHWAGANDHA: A medicinal herb classified as an "adaptogen" and said to reduce anxiety, cortisol, and blood sugar levels.

AVOCADO OIL: Obtained from the ripe fruit and expressed from the seed, this soothing oil is safe for sensitive skin.

BAKING SODA: An inorganic salt used as a buffering and neutralizing agent to soothe the skin. Also known as sodium bicarbonate.

BEE POLLEN: A tiny ball of pollen, saliva, and nectar or honey made by young bees when they land on flowers. It is a crunchy superfood known to relieve inflammation, boost immunity, reduce stress, and aid healing.

BEESWAX: An emulsifier for water and oil and often used in creams, balms, and waxes. White beeswax has been bleached to remove the otherwise natural yellow coloring.

BENTONITE CLAY: A noncomedogenic clay that regulates viscosity and absorbs water to create a gel-like consistency that removes toxins from the skin.

BROCCOLI SEED OIL: A moisturizing and anti-inflammatory oil that contains omega-3, omega-6, and omega-9 fatty acids, said to reduce skin conditions such as dermatitis, rosacea, and psoriasis.

BUTTERFLY PEA EXTRACT: Extracted from butterfly pea flowers, the butterfly pea is said to have brain-boosting effects with neurological benefits that help with depression, anxiety, and fever. Other potential benefits include improved eyesight, hair growth, and skin texture. It has also been traditionally used as an aphrodisiac.

CACAO: Derived from cacao beans, it contains polyphenols—naturally occurring antioxidants that have been linked to reduced inflammation, lower blood pressure, and improved cholesterol and blood sugar levels.

CALENDULA OIL: An oil that contains the botanical extract from the calendula blossom and said to have healing, antiseptic, and anti-inflammatory properties. Often used for oily or acne-prone skin.

CANDELILLA WAX: Obtained from candelilla plants and used to bind oils and waxes.

CARROT SEED OIL: Extracted from carrot seeds, it contains vitamin A and beta-carotene to treat dry, damaged skin.

CASTOR OIL: A carrier oil that easily penetrates the skin with high amounts of unsaturated fatty acids.

CHIA: These tiny black seeds are packed with nutrients (fiber, protein, calcium, magnesium, phosphorus) and antioxidants. Chia seed oil is very lush, with a creaminess that promotes glossy skin and hair.

CITRIC ACID: Derived from citrus fruits and used to stabilize products, adjust pH, and preserve formulation.

COCOA BUTTER: An edible fat extracted from cacao beans that undergoes some heating during the pressing. It softens the skin and easily liquefies at body temperature, making it easy to spread. *Cacao* butter is similar but is cold-pressed.

COCOA POWDER: Made by roasting crushed cacao beans after the fat is removed, it is rich in polyphenols (see Cacao) and known to reduce inflammation, increase blood flow, lower blood pressure, and improve cholesterol and blood sugar levels. *Cacao* powder is similar but is not processed at high temperatures and is considered raw.

COCONUT: Coconut water naturally occurs inside the coconut, while coconut milk is derived by crushing its flesh. Coconut powder is dehydrated coconut milk. Fractionated coconut oil, or MCT, is made when the long-chain fatty acids have been removed so the oil can no longer exist in a solid form. Fractionated coconut oil and coconut milk are known to be hydrating both inside and out.

COLLAGEN: Aids in reducing natural moisture loss through its ability to bind and retain many times its weight in water. Effective in skin moisturizers and in protecting the skin. Available in synthetically derived or bioengineered formulations.

CRANBERRY SEED OIL: Nourishing oil that contains vitamins A and E, and omegas-3, -6, and -9. It protects the skin's lipid barrier and promotes the absorption of fatty acids by the skin.

CUCUMBER SEED OIL: Cold pressed from the cleaned and dried seeds of premium quality cucumbers, it is then carefully filtered to obtain a brilliant, clear yellow oil with a mild, fresh cucumber aroma. With a high amount of phytosterols, it is known to support skin elasticity and maintain hydration.

CUPUAÇU BUTTER: Obtained from cupuaçu seeds in Brazil and used to create a thick, soft butter. Known to seal in moisture, it increases overall hydration, improves elasticity, and treats blemishes.

DISTILLED WATER: Purified water that has been boiled into vapor and condensed back into liquid in a separate container.

EMULSIFYING WAX: Unlike beeswax, this wax is vegan since it is a chemical mixture of emulsifiers and fatty alcohols.

ESSENTIAL OIL: An oil distilled from plants or other sources with a powerful fragrance and therapeutic benefits. Examples include sandalwood, palo santo, grapefruit, rose, and jasmine.

FRENCH GREEN CLAY: Originating from France, a natural bioorganic material that contains many valuable elements to clean pores, draw out impurities, and detoxify the skin.

GINGER: The powder derived from this root is known to aid digestion, treat nausea, and reduce pain and inflammation.

GRAPESEED OIL: Obtained by pressing grape seeds, its high linoleic acid and vitamin E content make it very moisturizing.

HEMP SEED OIL: Hemp seeds come from the hemp (*Cannabis sativa*) plant and are housed in small, brown hulls that are removed to reveal smaller, white seeds often called the hearts. Hemp seeds are rich in healthy fats, essential fatty acids, and proteins, but they contain no CBD. Hemp seed oil is dark green and easily absorbs into the skin. It is known to prevent dry skin and reduce acne without clogging pores.

HIBISCUS SEED OIL: Obtained from the seeds of the flower, this oil is rich in antioxidants like vitamin C and E and essential fatty acids and is known for its anti-aging properties.

HYALURONIC ACID: Maintains healthy skin by regulating water content, elasticity, and nutrient distribution. Its ability to retain water immediately smoothes rough skin and improves appearance.

HYDROSOL: Also known as flower waters, hydrosols are made by distilling botanicals. They are similar to essential oils but less concentrated and are often used as toners to revitalize the skin.

JOJOBA: As an oil, jojoba easily penetrates the skin and hair follicles and reduces moisture loss. Also available as esters, an emollient of jojoba oil and jojoba wax.

KAOLIN CLAY: Its ability to absorb excess oil and penetrate deep into pores makes it an ideal base for facial masks. It provides good coverage and adheres well to the skin but is easily removed with gentle cleansing.

KUKUI NUT OIL: Derived from Hawaiian kukui nuts and kernels that are roasted and then pressed for oil. Moisturizing and easily absorbed, the oil is ideal for chapped skin and irritation and often used to treat psoriasis and eczema.

MAGNESIUM FLAKES: A concentrated solution of magnesium chloride known to relax muscles by easing tension and stiffness.

MANGO BUTTER: Obtained from the kernel within the mango stone, it is an emollient with anti-inflammatory properties that may also promote cellular rejuvenation and protect against UV rays.

MANUKA HONEY: Produced in New Zealand and prized for its antibacterial properties and ability to heal wounds.

MARULA OIL: An emollient and humectant, it's high in antioxidants, essential fatty acids, and amino acids.

MATCHA: A powdered tea packed with antioxidants and said to boost metabolism, detoxify the skin, and enhance mood and concentration.

MICA: A series of ground silicate minerals that range in color and provide a glimmer or shimmer in formulations. Lab-created (versus naturally mined) is best as it avoids supporting unsatisfactory mining methods.

OLIVE OIL: Its great lubricity makes it a suitable carrier for essential oils and perfuming.

POMEGRANATE SEED OIL: A moisturizing and protective oil with soothing and anti-irritant properties known to be particularly beneficial for aging and sun-exposed skin. It contains vitamins B1, B2, and C as well as potassium and magnesium.

PUMPKIN SEED OIL: A skin-conditioning oil that can help improve the appearance of fine lines and wrinkles, skin tone, and elasticity.

RED RASPBERRY SEED OIL: Contains a high percentage of essential fatty acids, carotenoids, and vitamin E to condition the skin and protect against inflammation.

ROSE HIP OIL: Derived from the rose hips of various rose varietals, this emollient regulates oil-gland secretion and is known to heal wounds. Its moisture-retention abilities improve skin hydration.

SEA BUCKTHORN OIL: Extracted from a shrub native to Europe and Asia, this oil protects skin against harmful factors and contains high concentrations of vitamins C and E, carotenoids, amino acids, and flavonols.

SEA SALT: Its mildly abrasive crystals and health-enhancing minerals make it ideal for scrubs.

SHEA BUTTER: A natural fat obtained from the fruit of the African karite tree, this emollient alleviates dry skin and restores moisture with its anti-inflammatory properties.

SPIRULINA: A powder from blue-green algae that includes an excellent nutritional profile, including protein, vitamins B and E, carotenoids, iron, zinc, and copper. It has a hydrating effect on the skin and powerful antioxidant and anti-inflammatory properties.

SUNFLOWER SEED OIL: Expressed from sunflower seeds, this carrier oil softens and soothes the skin thanks to its high linoleic acid and essential fatty acid content.

SWEET ALMOND OIL: Obtained from sweet almonds that have been cleaned and crushed into a powder. The powder is then cold-pressed and filtered. The final product is very spreadable and, rich with vitamins E and A, moisturizing.

TEA TREE OIL: Distilling the leaves of tea trees produces an oil with a eucalyptus scent. The oil is a natural preservative with antiseptic and germicidal properties that promote healing, making it a popular topical remedy for fungi, infections, and skin disorders.

TURMERIC: This root and the spice ground from it is associated with healing, anti-inflammatory, and blood-purifying properties. It is used topically to treat eczema, rashes, acne, and other irritations.

VEGETABLE GLYCERIN: A clear, viscous liquid usually made from soybean, coconut, or palm oils. It keeps formulations from drying out and is said to increase skin hydration and decrease irritation.

WITCH HAZEL: Derived from the bark and leaves of a North American shrub, it's excellent as a natural toner and also typically added to formulations at a dose of 2 to 5 percent to treat burns, irritations, insect bites, and bruises.

ZINC OXIDE: Obtained from zinc ore, a commonly found mineral, to protect against ultraviolet rays—both UVA and UVB—with astringent, antiseptic, and antibacterial properties. The FDA has approved zinc oxide as a safe and effective sunscreen.

CBD Industry Terms

AERIAL PLANT PARTS: The entirety of the plant above the soil, including leaves, stems, flowers, fruits, and seeds. Used in most full-spectrum oils.

BIOAVAILABILITY: A subcategory of absorption. The degree and the rate at which a compound is absorbed by the body's circulatory system. A medication administered intravenously has a bioavailability of 100 percent.

BROAD SPECTRUM: Regarding hemp extract, this type of oil has many of hemp's naturally occurring compounds and cannabinoids but does not contain THC.

CANNABIDIOL (CBD): A nonintoxicating cannabinoid found in cannabis that has many potential therapeutic benefits, including anti-inflammatory, analgesic, anti-anxiety, and seizure-prevention properties.

CANNABINOIDS: Active compounds found in cannabis, including CBD, THC, and many others.

CANNABINOL (CBN): A nonpsychoactive (i.e., won't get you high) compound created when THC ages.

CANNABIS: The name of the plant genus that includes both marijuana and hemp.

CB1 AND CB2 RECEPTORS: G-protein coupled cannabinoid receptors in humans that can be found in the peripheral nervous system and central nervous system. CBD binds to these receptors to influence your endocannabinoid system.

CERTIFICATE OF ANALYSIS (COA): A document issued by a regulatory or quality-assurance entity (often a lab) that verifies the adherence to product specifications and standards of production of certain products, such as food and drugs. Specific to CBD, a COA will confirm the potency (total milligrams and percentage of each cannabinoid) and purity of the product to ensure that it contains no pesticides, herbicides, heavy metals, or solvents.

CO_2 EXTRACTION: A process that uses pressurized carbon dioxide to pull the desired compounds from a plant. This extraction process creates a light-amber-colored oil that can be consumed by vaping (see disclaimer on page 24), applying sublingually or topically, or ingesting orally.

EDIBLE: A cannabis or hemp extract–infused product that is ingested, usually in the form of a drink or bite-size snack.

ENDOCANNABINOID SYSTEM: A biological system composed of endocannabinoids, which are endogenous lipid-based retrograde neurotransmitters. This system is responsible for influencing mood, appetite, memory, and inflammation.

ENTOURAGE EFFECT: A mechanism by which active plant compounds act synergistically with one another to boost the medicinal benefits of cannabis.

FULL SPECTRUM: In regard to hemp extract, an oil that has all of hemp's naturally occurring compounds and cannabinoids. None have been removed during the extraction process so that they mutually benefit one another.

HEMP: A variety of cannabis that has served a wide range of purposes for more than ten thousand years. Hemp fibers can be used to create items such as paper, clothing, fabric, rope, and building materials. Hemp contains less than 0.3 percent THC in the United States.

HEMP SEED OIL: Also known as *Cannabis sativa* seed oil, this oil is extracted from the seeds of a hemp plant and does not contain CBD.

INDICA: A subspecies of the cannabis plant with short stems and broad leaves, characterized as having a more relaxing effect than sativa.

INGESTIBLE: A form of cannabis or hemp extract that is taken orally.

ISOLATE: Regarding hemp extract, this type of oil contains only the cannabinoid CBD. No other beneficial compounds of the hemp plant are found in isolate.

LIMONENE: A colorless liquid terpene hydrocarbon with a lemon-like scent, it's present in lemon oil, orange oil, and many other essential oils, as well as cannabis.

LINALOOL: A fragrant liquid terpene found in many essential oils used to create perfumes, soaps, and flavorings. It occurs naturally in cannabis plants with a smell similar to sweet lavender with a touch of citrus.

MACRODOSE: A very large amount of a compound used to test its maximum effects or benefits.

MARIJUANA: A variety of the cannabis plant that is grown and used mainly for its psychoactive effects.

MICRODOSE: A very small amount of a compound used to test for or benefit from its physiological action while minimizing undesirable side effects.

MYRCENE: A liquid terpene hydrocarbon and a significant essential oil in several plants, including cannabis and hops.

PHYTOCANNABINOID: Naturally occurring cannabinoids found in the cannabis plant. *Phyto* is a prefix that means "pertaining to or derived from plants."

PINENE: A colorless liquid terpene found in turpentine, juniper oil, and other natural extracts. It's also found in cannabis plants.

PSYCHOACTIVE: Affecting the mind or behavior.

SATIVA: A tall, lanky subspecies of the cannabis plant characterized as having uplifting and energetic effects.

SUBLINGUAL: Situated or applied under the tongue. This ingestion method achieves peak blood levels within ten to fifteen minutes, which is generally much faster than oral ingestion. The bioavailability of this ingestion method is also generally higher than oral.

TERPENE: A large and diverse class of organic compounds, produced by a variety of plants, often having a strong odor to protect the plants by deterring herbivores and attracting predators and parasites of herbivores.

TERPINOLENE: A liquid terpene found in essential oils and cannabis recognizable for its woodsy aroma in tandem with citrus and floral notes.

THC: Tetrahydrocannabinol, a crystalline compound that is the main active ingredient in marijuana.

THCA: Tetrahydrocannabinolic acid, a non-intoxicating cannabinoid found in freshly picked and living cannabis. As cannabis dries, THCA slowly converts to THC.

THIRD-PARTY TESTING: Indicates that an independent organization or entity has tested and produced unbiased details—in the form of a COA—of the product being reviewed.

TINCTURE: A liquid form of a supplement, often medicinal and usually in a dropper bottle, which also contains a carrier oil.

TOLERANCE: The capacity of the body to endure or become less responsive to a substance with repeated use or exposure.

TOPICAL: A product designed to be placed directly on the surface of the skin.

TRANSDERMAL: Relating to the application of a medicine or drug through the skin, typically by using an adhesive patch so that it is absorbed slowly into the body over time.

VAPE: An electronic device that allows the user to inhale and exhale vapor of cannabis oil or flower. See disclaimer on page 24.

WATER-SOLUBLE: Able to be dissolved in water. Water-soluble vitamins, such as C and B complex, are carried into the tissues but not stored in the body, unlike fat-soluble vitamins A, D, E, and K, which are absorbed along with fats in the diet and can be stored in fatty tissue.

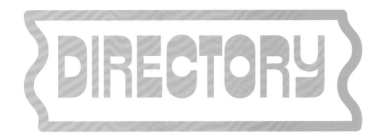

Cosmetic Ingredients and Botanicals

BRAMBLE BERRY: Offers a large selection of cosmetic bases and oils along with other specialty ingredients and materials (bottles, molds, tools, etc.).
⊕ *BrambleBerry.com*

DANDELION BOTANICAL COMPANY: An apothecary offering a wide range of herbs, spices, salts, and essential oils.
⊕ *DandelionBotanical.com*

DOTERRA: Specializes in therapeutic-grade essential oils and oil blends.
⊕ *DoTERRA.com*

FROM NATURE WITH LOVE: Offers a large selection of cosmetic ingredients, such as sugars, salts, oils, and powders. They also carry cookware, molds, and various packaging supplies.
⊕ *FromNaturewithLove.com*

MAKING COSMETICS: Carries bulk ingredients as well as kits, samples, containers, and cosmetic bases for customization.
⊕ *MakingCosmetics.com*

MOUNTAIN ROSE HERBS: Offers bulk herbs, spices, clays, butters, and oils. They pride themselves on product quality, sustainable packaging, fair-trade practices, and watershed conservation.
⊕ *MountainRoseHerbs.com*

Grocery and Specialty Foods

AMAZON: Often called the "everything store," Amazon is a great place to source containers and packaging, such as jars, dropper bottles, molds, or muslin bags.
⊕ *Amazon.com*

CAP BEAUTY: Features a grocery section dedicated to unique adaptogens, superfoods, and pantry staples.
⊕ *CAPBeauty.com*

EREWHON MARKET: Organic grocery that strives to provide ethically and sustainably produced products.
⊕ *ErewhonMarket.com*

GOLDE: Offers superfood essentials such as turmeric and matcha.
⊕ *Golde.co*

KAUAI FARMACY: Produces spices, honey, herbal tinctures, and superfoods on the Hawaiian island of Kauai.
⊕ *KauaiFarmacy.com*

LASSENS NATURAL FOODS & VITAMINS: Offers 100-percent organic produce and low-processed, additive-free foods.
⊕ *Lassens.com*

MOON JUICE: Creates their own adaptogenic blends and plant proteins.
⊕ *MoonJuice.com*

SUN POTION: Offers organically and fairly sourced nutritional supplements and superfoods.
⊕ *SunPotion.com*

THRIVE MARKET: A membership-based market offering organic, non-GMO, and sustainable grocery items.
⊕ *ThriveMarket.com*

TRADER JOE'S: Offers its own brand of grocery items without artificial flavors, preservatives, or genetically modified ingredients.
⊕ *TraderJoes.com*

WHOLE FOODS MARKET: Has a wide selection of grocery items free of hydrogenated fats and artificial colors, flavors, and preservatives. Locations throughout the United States and Canada.
⊕ *WholeFoodsMarket.com*

CBD Products and Education

DAZEY CBD: That's us! We offer full-spectrum CBD oil and CBD-infused skin care.
🌐 *ShopDazey.com*

FLEUR MARCHÉ: Curated online CBD marketplace founded by two Goop alumni.
🌐 *FleurMarche.com*

KITCHEN TOKE: CBD marketplace and cannabis-infused cooking resource with digital and print publications.
🌐 *KitchenToke.com*

MISS GRASS: This online magazine and cannabis shop offers CBD products and lifestyle items.
🌐 *MissGrass.com*

POPLAR: An online marketplace that offers a curated assortment of CBD products.
🌐 *Shop-Poplar.com*

STANDARD DOSE: A retailer that offers plant-based and CBD products both online and at their store in Manhattan, New York.
🌐 *StandardDose.com*

SVN SPACE: Hemp-focused media brand with an online store offering CBD and lifestyle products.
🌐 *SvnSpace.com*

WHITE LABEL CBD MARKET: Curated online CBD marketplace that evaluates each product with a proprietary process.
🌐 *Shop-WhiteLabel.com*

Cannabis and CBD Organizations

American Herbal Products Association
🌐 *AHPA.org*

Hemp Industries Association
🌐 *TheHIA.org*

Leafly
🌐 *Leafly.com*

National Cannabis Industry Association
🌐 *TheCannabisIndustry.org*

Project CBD
🌐 *ProjectCBD.org*

Realm of Caring
🌐 *RealmofCaring.org*

UCLA Cannabis Research Initiative
🌐 *UCLAHealth.org/Cannabis*

US Hemp Authority
🌐 *USHempAuthority.org*

US Hemp Roundtable
🌐 *HempSupporter.com*

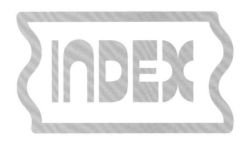

INDEX

Note: Page numbers in *italic* refer to photographs.

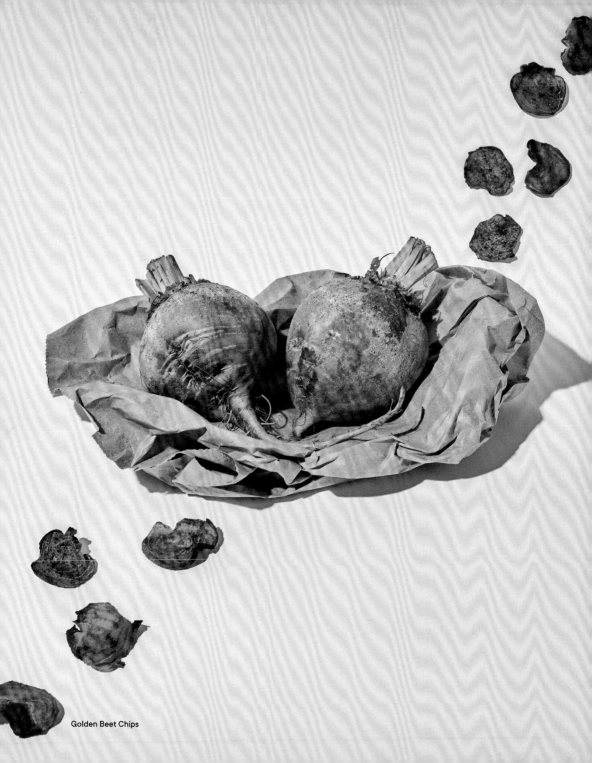

Golden Beet Chips

Printed in China

SASQUATCH BOOKS with colophon is a registered trademark of Penguin Random House LLC

24 23 22 21 20   9 8 7 6 5 4 3 2 1

Editor: Jen Worick

Production editor: Bridget Sweet

Designer: Tony Ong

Nail art: Kayla Wakayama

Hand models: Tori Bodin, Emily Hoeke, and Cortnee Blayton

Interior illustrations: Tony Ong

Photographs: Lauren Segal

Food and prop styling: Mandy Kehoe

Dazey brand design: Emily Hoeke and Scott Schwarz

The author and publisher have made every effort to ensure that the information in this book was correct at press time.

Library of Congress Cataloging-in-Publication Data
Names: Bodin, Tori, author. | Tarello, Chris, author.
Title: CBD & chill : 75 self-care recipes for everyday wellness / Tori
   Bodin and Chris Tarello.
Other titles: CBD and chill
Description: Seattle : Sasquatch Books, [2020] | Includes index.
Identifiers: LCCN 2019052852 (print) | LCCN 2019052853 (ebook) | ISBN
   9781632173195 (hardcover) | ISBN 9781632173201 (ebook)
Subjects: LCSH: Cooking (Marijuana) | LCGFT: Cookbooks.
Classification: LCC TX819.M25 B64 2020 (print) | LCC TX819.M25 (ebook) |
   DDC 641.6/379–dc23
LC record available at https://lccn.loc.gov/2019052852
LC ebook record available at https://lccn.loc.gov/2019052853

ISBN: 978-1-63217-319-5

Sasquatch Books
1904 Third Avenue, Suite 710
Seattle, WA 98101
SasquatchBooks.com

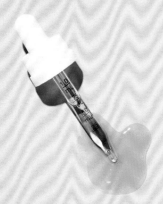

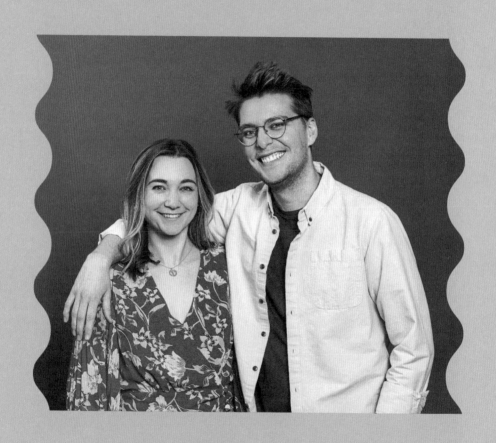